YOU HAVE
THE POWER

WHY DIDN'T MY DOCTOR
TELL ME ABOUT THIS?

By   Dr Michael Elstein

Written & Published by Dr. Michael Elstein

Copyright Dr. Michael Elstein 2005

Design & Illustrations by Aliart
aliart.a@bigpond.net.au

Cover Design by character

Printed and bound in Australia

ISBN: 0-646-45123-5

IN MEMORIUM:

BENNIE 5/11/1991-13/11/2004

YOUR SPIRIT WILL NEVER DIE

ACKNOWLEDGMENTS

I would like to thank Charles, Alice

and my mother Jacqueline

for their tireless commitment

to bringing this book to print.

CONTENTS

Dr Michael Elstein is a medical and health visionary, being a pioneer and a member of the "Wellness Evolution" that started in the late 1990's, Michael has now been propelled into the 21st Century by the desire to feel good about his past achievements and is always seeking to achieve higher standards within his programmes.

Michael is one of the doctors who, in the 1980's, saw the failures of the medical system and had the courage to change his practices for the benefit of his patients. This was at a time when doctors could be punished severely for not practicing the drug-based medicine they were taught. Michael not only had the courage and intellectual honesty to change, he had the tenacity to continue improving his methods of health care in a hostile medical environment which persists today. Doctors have been trained to look for and measure pathological states and treat them with drugs, surgery or radiation, the cut, burn or poison modalities.

However, there is overwhelming evidence that lifestyle changes including exercise, diet, vitamins, herbs, meditation, music, art and even pets can reduce the incidence and severity of many of our killer diseases and may, if appropriately used, even reverse them. That's why Michael has written this book, and that's why this book is so important to you, and the rest of Australia.

The current crisis in Australia's healthcare system requires the adoption of healthcare policies that embrace natural healthcare, are based on a wellness system of health optimisation, the prevention of disease, and empower consumers to take greater responsibility for their health. This book can show the way out of this crisis.

Consumers have increasingly chosen natural healthcare products. Approximately 80% of Australian GPs are referring patients for complementary healthcare treatments.

Australians spend approximately $1.5 billion in consumer dollars on natural healthcare products, excluding services. Dr Michael's book contains information that will raise the wellness of Australians and save the Government money.

Current health policy in Australia focuses on the treatment of disease as opposed to the prevention of disease and optimisation of health. The "drug and disease" paradigm is costly, not only in monetary terms but also the human toll of pain and suffering, and the impact on productivity and quality of life. We need a Department of Health Optimisation which will employ the wellness practices in this book.

Mainstream medical professionals are trained to think and act in terms of disease. Prevention is a secondary consideration in most medical schools and practices, and true health optimisation in this context is almost non-existent. According to conventional medical leaders, the main achievements in the prevention of disease have been anti-smoking campaigns, encouragement of exercise and vaccination. This shows our most eminent scientists admitting that, despite everything we know about the causes of chronic illness, we have not been successful in the promotion of good nutrition. Of these 'successful' campaigns, only exercise could really be considered a health promotion activity. Michael's approach to the empowerment of individual's as outlined in this book, goes much further than the orthodox thinking about health and will significantly contribute to the "wellbeing literature" available to the Australian public.

The escalating costs of healthcare in Australia were

clearly outlined in the 2002-03 Federal Budget, which included an Intergenerational Report describing the future impact of an ageing population on Commonwealth finances. Now is the time to act to integrate natural healthcare treatments into our disease-focused system. To do this requires appropriate recognition by government, the media and the community for the valuable contribution natural healthcare products and services make to the real health of Australians.

The current minister for Health, Tony Abbott is in favour of the "Wellness Model" approach to health, stating it is far preferable for people to seek natural healthcare products over synthetic drugs wherever possible. The "Wellness Model" of health works in accordance with prevention, in that people are given the necessary tools and encouragement in order to maximise their health status and prevent illness. It also emphasises the importance of striving for optimal health achievement even in patients with severe disease or chronic illness.

Health is not merely the absence of disease. Our entire system of healthcare is devoted to the idea that you wait until you get a disease, then you choose a drug to "fix" it. The other alternatives in mainstream medicine are surgery, radiotherapy or "wait and see". Healthcare should be more than that and optimum health should be the objective of everyone. In the end it is cheaper to achieve health than spend on disease care, and we spend a lot of time and money getting ill and diseased. The killer diseases, like heart disease, cancer, stroke, diabetes, depression and asthma, are, in many cases, the culmination of years of effort.

Let us look at some examples of health promotion activities that are safe, proven and effective in terms of pro-actively caring for our health. Firstly, consider heart disease, our number one killer. Many Australians take statin drugs, the recognised mainstream way to reduce cholesterol. A common scenario goes like this; middle aged Australian male is prescribed statins for high cholesterol. The statins, in blocking the metabolic pathways that make cholesterol, also block the production of an important energy regulator Coenzyme Q10. Low Coenzyme Q10 levels cause an increase in blood pressure, and a weakening of the heart muscle. The long-term prognosis for our patient is therefore not good, because the underlying causes and nutritional factors have not been adequately addressed.

Instead, if men at risk of heart disease used the CHC treatments of an exercise regime, fish oils, plant sterols and dietary changes, high cholesterol levels could be brought down gradually and safely, without the side effects of drug therapy. A further question that needs to be asked is: Why do 44% of American cardiologists take vitamins C and E themselves, but they don't routinely recommend them for their patients.

Another condition that contributes enormously to the cost of disease care in this country is arthritis, yet this is a disease that responds extremely well to diet, and diet therapy has the potential to save the disease budget millions of dollars. Simply prescribing drugs fails to address the cause of the problem, and the failure to address causative factors results in more disease. Scandinavian doctors commonly recommend dietary changes for arthritis sufferers more fish, fruit and vegetables, and less sugar, fat and dairy. Added to this an antioxidant regime including the vitamins A, C and E, and the minerals zinc, selenium and copper, together with more fish oils and exercise, and the results are outstanding. With the recent concerns over the Cox2 Inhibitors causing more strokes and heart attacks, the public have turned toward a natural molecule called glucosamine for its anti-arthritic effects and cartilage regeneration, without serious side effects. These approaches not only helps arthritis, it reduces the incidence of other chronic diseases later, increases the productivity and wellbeing of the individual and saves the government millions of dollars.

Michael also, early in his book, addresses the issue of obesity and overweight, almost a pandemic in western industrialized nations.

The Obesity epidemic, whilst being a non-issue for many politicians, some even contending that it is non-existent, is a catastrophic failure of our public health authorities, government and health professionals to act appropriately over two decades ago when the problems first became evident. Obesity and many other health problems we now face, was predicted over 25 years ago and the authorities ignored us. In fact, the medical and nutrition professions continued on the promotion of disease road by not only ignoring us, but by embracing the sugar industry with all its metabolic ramifications and the fast food industry, as being important parts of a "balanced" Australian diet. The damage has been done. Three generations of Australians are affected by overweight or obesity.

The damage will continue long into the future. I now predict that the dozen or so serious degenerative diseases highly associated with obesity, overweight will become more sinister and the cancers related to fatness, poor diet and sedentary living will become even more malignant. Why? The biochemistry tells us so. And the medicalised expensive disease care system we call a health system, will not cope. There won't be the trained human resources or the money to do it. The trends are happening now. We have a doctor shortage and the hospitals are straining at the seams. The Pharmaceutical Benefits Scheme has exceeded $6 billion per annum. Only 5 years ago, it was just over $3 billion. This is absolutely unsustainable.

Michael's book looks at the disease process from the viewpoint of its biochemical causes, the first changes that we are aware of on the downhill slide to degenerative disease. He takes us logically and clearly through the various stages of highly rational wellness programs for a variety of serious conditions. He supports his practices with evidence that is appropriate. Michael's personal touches to his clinical authorship are matched by his art-and-science of patient histories. Always meaningful and always looking for the fundamental biochemical "lesion" requiring correction. His messages are those messages which frequently hold public audiences spellbound, messages about natural health and what the individual can do for themselves. These are the messages that should be taken to the highest offices in the country, the messages that politicians and bureaucrats need to act on. The book should be read by the sick, the unwell and everyone who wants to feel good and stay that way.

BY PROFESSOR IAN BRIGHTHOPE

President of the Australian College of Nutritional and Environmental Medicine

Dr Michael Elstein is the CEO of a vitamin company called Neozest which has released Memozeal a formulation designed to enhance memory and help manage tinnitus. Two new formulations, Oxyzeal, an antioxidant designed to prevent heart disease and Flavozeal, an anti-inflammatory are planned for release in 2006.

CHAPTER 1

You have the POWER

This book is about health, vitality, fun and joy. It's also about passion, power and purpose. Wouldn't it be wonderful if you were supercharged with energy, joy and passion and these occupied a major part of your day? Sadly I don't know many people who are brimming with health, whose days are filled with joy and who are passionately driven to pursue their goals.

I believe that it is possible to turn this all around. This is not a dream. It is achievable and it could be your reality. As good health lies at the very core of our existence, I've devoted a major segment of this book to describing how this can be achieved. I'm writing this book to help you to be healthy, stay healthy and not get sick. Health is the essence of all functioning. If you aren't healthy you simply cannot operate. But it is the power that drives you. Finding your power will help you to discover your passion and once you harness your power and your passion you will become an irresistible force. You will then understand why you are on this planet. Each and every one of us has this power, we all have passion and we all have purpose, it's just a matter of uncovering that power and that passion and that purpose. Once you feel powerful everything else will flow. So many of us have not accessed the power, we don't understand it and we are pursuing this elusive yet awesome quality incorrectly. You see the funny thing is that you already have the power.

You have within you the capacity to be the most powerful, passionate committed person that you have ever known. You have the power to make a massive contribution to the health and wellbeing of this planet. We are all here to be equally powerful, to appreciate each other's power and to get along in a mutually loving and caring way. Imagine what the world would be like if this were the case, if we were all powerful people executing our daily activities in the most effective and caring fashion, if each and every one of us was the best at what we did and we did this lovingly. Let me explain.

Recently I presented a 5-minute talk about the anti-ageing programme that I offer at a business meeting which I frequent every week in the city. This is a meeting attended by business people from all walks of life, the purpose being to introduce ourselves, network with the other attendees, receive a 5-minute speech by one of the members about themselves or their business and then hear a motivational speaker, usually someone telling us how we can become more successful and wealthier in our business endeavours. At this meeting a microphone is passed around the room and each of us has a turn to stand up, say who we are and what we do and tell the attendees how they can benefit from our services. We then proceed to give a thought of the day. You can imagine that this would be a somewhat unnerving experience leading to a certain modicum of anxiety. Like everyone else I accomplished this ordeal with a reasonable amount of aplomb and when everyone had finished stepped up for my longer speech to discuss the benefits of the anti-ageing programme. I had prepared this speech at home and even in rehearsal it didn't seem to flow. For some reason I wasn't able to tap into the purpose and the passion that I felt about this programme and my presentation lacked fire and commitment. I thought that once I stood in front of the audience everything would change.

How wrong I was. The talk was far too cerebral, there was way too much information and I started to get caught up in the content rather than conveying the essence of the message. Instead of telling them that I have a health programme that is second to none I started to give detailed examples of patients I had successfully treated. After 5 minutes I was only ½ way through my talk yet the president of the club proceeded to indicate that I should finish. I immediately became tongue-tied thinking that he had picked up the mood of the others and that they weren't really interested in what I had to say. I quickly thanked the audience and sat down feeling utterly embarrassed and demolished. Various members of the audience come up to congratulate me afterwards but I knew that I had tanked. Fortunately I knew the motivational speaker and I requested that he provide me with a critique of my talk. He indicated that my talk was far too detailed and that I needed to keep it simple and stick with one example at most.

They say that huge pain can provide profound lessons for all of us. I would have to say that this experience was a major turning point in my life. I came home and thought about my presentation and realised that it lacked passion. I wasn't communicating to the audience the essence of my message: that I would provide them with the most comprehensive, the best health assessment that they could obtain anywhere in the universe. Have you ever tried saying that you are the best? Have you ever tried saying that there is absolutely no one else better than you, no one anywhere? Do you remember who was the first to do this? Muhammad Ali was the first to say, 'I am the greatest' and didn't we love him for it. When you can say with total conviction that you have the best knowledge and skills with regard to your chosen vocation and that you can provide the most compassionate service then you too might discover what it means to have the power. You might find that your whole body resonates with passion and fire. And then miraculously you will understand why you are here. Your mission on this planet will become clear. You might think that I'm encouraging you to be arrogant but you might actually find that this is a very humbling experience. Once your self-doubt starts to evaporate you might find that you are more confident, open-hearted, loving and joyous in all your interactions.

When you manifest your power magic might happen. Let me tell you what I mean. The other night I had to go to a meeting in a part of the city that I had only been to once before. I was vaguely sure of the location so I drove to that part of the city and then stopped at a corner store and went inside so that I could view the roadmap that I was trying to decipher with difficulty. When I went into the store a gentleman behind the counter asked me what I was looking for and I indicated the name of the street to which he casually replied that it was just down the hill. I got back in my car and drove down the hill and lo and behold there it was. Without much effort I had found the place. After this meeting I had to drive to the house of good friends of mine to get a dinner suit that I was borrowing for a ball on Saturday night. They had just moved house and I had only been there once before. Like the previous venue I had some idea where they lived but couldn't remember the name of street. I drove to that part of the city and followed another car taking a turn into a side street off the street which I was on. I looked at the name of the street as I made this turn and there it was: the exact street I wanted. Once again I had reached my destination with ease. The next day I went into a fruit shop to purchase some fruit and vegetables. The purchase came to $13.25. I took out three five-dollar notes and the store owner enquired whether I had the exact change. I took back one of the five dollar notes and reached into my wallet, grabbed hold of some change and placed it on the counter. The amount came to exactly $3.25. I had wanted to find a gardener to look after the front and back garden of my unit as it was looking rather shabby and unkempt and I just didn't have the time to devote to this. I hadn't seen the gardener who tends to the grounds that surround the townhouse complex in which I live for over one year. When I returned to my townhouse that day there he was just outside my unit going about his daily duties ready and available to do the work I needed. I wanted to update my website and needed to find someone who could do the job in the most professional way. I went to another one of those networking business meetings, sat down to prepare for the speaker of the day and the first person to come and sit at my table was a pleasant young gentleman called Endo who handed me his business card. Endo's business just so happened to be involved with updating websites.

Now these all might be coincidences and these aren't major events which are going to shape the future of mankind but I still think there is something significant and magical going on here. When you have discovered the power, when your life is headed in the direction of your divine purpose then you don't have to expand that much effort, you will be directed and guided to your destiny. Over the past two weeks I have been eating less. I just haven't needed that much food. I have needed to lose a few kilos to get down to my ideal weight and have achieved this with ease. Have you ever found that the more you try to lose weight, the harder it is and the more difficult it becomes? Life should not be a struggle. It only becomes a struggle when you become too attached to wealth and success.

Now don't get me wrong. I'm not saying you should not pursue these qualities. If your goals are to acquire wealth and to be successful or you have already attained these then hats off to you. These aspirations are indeed commendable. However I would caution you about becoming too caught up in the never-ending pursuit of desires that may ultimately consume your soul. I just don't believe that chasing wealth and success will truly empower you or really make you happy. There are many men who think that wealth and success will give them power and make them attractive to the opposite sex. This might be true in a superficial fashion but I don't believe it will lead to really fulfilling relationships. True power is associated with humility. The experience of true power leads to acts of loving-kindness, to a state of being able to listen and receive with an open heart and the capacity to say; 'I'm here to help and love you.' This is what really relating is all about. You don't need wealth and success to experience this kind of relationship. In fact wealth and success will get in the way. If you are attractive because you have wealth and success what will happen when you don't have these? How much wealth and success will you need to make you appear powerful? Real power will arrive when you discover your passion and your purpose and you realise why you are here. Life becomes easy and effortless once you have this power. Life is not about endless chasing, endless struggling. Real power will guide you effortlessly. Yes, we are limitless. We are limitless because we aren't really separate. Love is the limitless energy which we can experience once we have full access to the power.

In essence we are on this planet to be healthy, vital, loving human beings helping each other get along. There is so much wealth in acts of loving-kindness. Love is so simple. Just telling someone you love them, giving them a hug, smiling at them when they serve you in the supermarket, that is what love is all about. These simple acts can make your day very rich and fill your heart till it's overflowing. If we were to help and love each other would there be a need to fight, to be constantly irritated and angry, to hold on to resentments, to drive each other off the road because of uncontrollable rage? Would there be a need to control, dominate or invade? Dare I say it but would there even be a need for war?

What a wonderful world it would be if we all were tremendously powerful, passionate and loving. Think what we could achieve, how many people we could help, how we could use the money we earn to assist those in need. This book is about discovering your power and becoming the healthiest person you can be. What would our lives be like if we woke to greet the day and each other with wonder, excitement and appreciation. 'Wow, it's great to be alive and I'm so glad you are here.' Yes my dear reader it is.

chapter 2

Medicine's Future

Health is such a precious gift. It reverberates at the very centre of our being. Then again what is health? Do you want to be healthier? Are you concerned about your health? Many of us only start to take action when we aren't healthy, when we become unwell, sometimes so unwell that tragically there is not much that can be done. This is human nature, to fix things when they have become broken. I'm hoping that this book will change that.

You might be wondering what the 'this' is in the title. 'This' stands for health, energy and vitality and the tests you can undergo which will enlighten you as to what is getting in the way of you enjoying robust health. The reason your doctor isn't concerned about these things is because (with all due respects to your doctor) he or she is not too concerned about health. Doctors aren't trained to promote health. They are trained to treat sickness, which is a shame. Wouldn't it be better to know how to keep your body healthy than to patch it up when it gets sick? That's what this book is all about: keeping your body healthy. You are about to be provided with information that will change your life. You see I'm an anti-ageing and weight loss physician. I help people to prevent and delay the ageing process as much as this is possible and I help people to prevent the diseases of ageing such as heart disease, Parkinson's and Alzheimer's disease as well as cancer. I also help people to effectively lose weight particularly those people who are finding this extremely difficult. The truth is we are all ageing and as we age many of us will put on weight. This is natural. It's natural to age and yes it's also natural to put on weight as you age at least till you reach the age of sixty. Nature wants us to age. Once you have reached your biological use-by date and you have procreated then nature is going to wave you goodbye. Nature doesn't want you to hang around. And nature doesn't mind if you gain weight.

Now, let me tell you about the world we live in. We live in a culture which values three qualities extremely highly: youthfulness, beauty and slimness. This is especially true for women. Our culture tells us that if you are young, slim and beautiful you have the power and you can get whatever you want. If you were to open up any women's magazine and you were to take a look at any of the advertisements that assault your eyes page after page after page you'll find beautiful young women adorned in an array of garments or bedecked in the gaudiest jewellery exhorting you to do one thing: to purchase what those perfect young models are wearing. They want you to race out and buy that dress, hurry to your nearest store and acquire that jewellery. The reason for this is simple. If you were to wear what they are wearing then you can be that woman and if you can be that woman then you too can have whatever you want. Our culture says: 'be young, slim and beautiful' and nature says: 'no can do.' Nature says: ' sorry, you are going to get old and then you are going to shuffle off this mortal coil.' This is the bitter pill that we have to swallow.

So let me give you the good news before you get too depressed. Here's the antidote. As I said before I'm an anti-ageing doctor. Every day in my medical practice I help my patients to regain their youthful exuberance. I help my patients to rediscover their spark, their enthusiasm, that fire in the belly that says: 'I can do this.' You don't necessarily have to be that young woman in the advertisement to rediscover your power and your lost youth. We are the baby boomer generation. We want to carry on forever. We don't want to age. I'm on your side, I too covet eternal health. I also want to remain youthful for as long as I can. Sadly there are many people out there who have lost their youthfulness. Every day I treat patients who are exhausted, depressed, stressed, can't lose weight, aren't getting enough sleep and who look old beyond their years. What I do is help change all this.

When I saw Howard a 58 year-old accountant for the first time his physical fortunes had taken a marked nosedive. He had precious little energy, wasn't sleeping well and endured annoying persistent ringing in both ears. Whatever he tried he wasn't able to successfully lose weight. He suffered from restricted movement in his right shoulder and his memory was going downhill rapidly. This was a man who used to do a 5km jog quite comfortably, could easily do 20 push-ups without a break and had a mind which was as sharp as a tack. Seemingly overnight he had become a basket case with no drive, no enthusiasm and the only desire he had was to take a load off in front of the television after a hard day's work. Quite rapidly he appeared to be deteriorating into an ageing, unattractive couch potato with no passion for his job or his wife. He was about to throw in the towel thinking with abject resignation that this was what ageing was all about and there was nothing that he could do about it. I was his last resort.

It's been one year since that initial consultation and Howard has undergone a remarkable transformation. His energy and vitality are the best he has experienced in the past ten years. He's lost weight, has returned to his 5km jog and his right shoulder is functioning without any restriction. The ringing sensation in his ear hardly troubles him and his sleep patterns are much improved. How did we achieve this magical reformation? How was Howard able to turn his life around so dramatically? What he needed was a total health package. Once his hormonal levels and vitamin status were assessed along with his other nutrients and we found out that he was deficient in some of these vital substances he commenced a programme specific to his needs and imbalances that over time made Howard the kind of dynamo that he used to be. He has remained on his hormones, which include testosterone, thyroid hormone and dehydroepiandrosterone (DHEA) as well as an assortment of vitamins and nutrients and because he feels so well nothing is going to deter him from sticking with this regimen.

Helen who is 72 and remains in full employment as the local school librarian is another case in point. She's been taking hormones since she commenced menopause at the age of 51 and has been on vitamins and other supplements for the past ten years. Ask the other younger members of her gym who find it difficult to keep up with her and they all think that she is in her early sixties. If you think ageing is all about becoming flabby, fatigued, mentally incapacitated and dysfunctional and there's nothing you can do about it then I'm here to tell you that the experience I have with my patients is exactly the opposite. The patients I see are sick and tired of being sick and tired and they want to do something about it.

This is a phenomenon that I've encountered many times in my practice. I see so many people who make considerable shifts once they commence the appropriate hormone and vitamin programme, start the diet that suits their individual needs and improve the function of their adrenal glands, liver and digestive systems. It's that simple. Nothing gives me more joy than to help my patients to become youthful, energised and mentally rejuvenated. There is nothing more rewarding than seeing my patients healthy and happy. Time and again I have found that hormone and vitamin treatments are an integral part of this process.

You might be wondering how I can be so enthusiastic about the benefits of hormones when recent evidence suggests that these chemicals might do us more harm than good.

This concern has been fuelled by the much publicised 'Women's Health Initiative' (WHI) study which set out to prove that hormone replacement therapy (HRT) provides women with a healthy passage through the ageing process and demonstrable protection against the diseases of ageing such as heart disease, dementia, cancer and osteoporosis. Instead the results of this study appeared to deliver the kind of results that the supporters of HRT didn't anticipate with evidence that the risk for breast cancer and heart disease actually increased although the incidence of bowel cancer and osteoporosis enjoyed a downward trend. The overall conclusion from this study was that HRT could not be endorsed as a long-term strategy to keep women healthy and to prevent age-related diseases.

However, once the dust settled and the experts started to examine the facts in a critical fashion, it became abundantly clear that the WHI trial was flawed in many ways. The average age of the women who undertook this experiment was 63. This is not the usual time when HRT is initiated. It's customary to commence HRT soon after menopause around the age of 50 and studies have in fact shown that women who do this are likely to derive the most benefits in terms of preventing osteoporosis, dementia and heart disease. (1) Once this window of opportunity that exists in early menopause is lost then embarking on a course of HRT at a later stage will be far less beneficial.

There are two major female hormones - oestrogen and progesterone. The form of HRT that the women in this trial received included Premarin, which is oestrogen derived from the urine of a horse and Provera, a type of progesterone formulation called a progestogen, that actually has a different chemical structure when compared with the natural progesterone manufactured in the female body. It is widely acknowledged in the medical community that Premarin and Provera are just about the unsafest forms of HRT that you can find. A metabolic by-product of Premarin called equilenin, which circulates in the female body, has been found to damage DNA. Provera has been associated with the promotion of heart disease, stroke and possibly breast cancer. That a group of expert physicians in the USA chose to use this form of HRT is frankly astonishing. If you then administer this treatment to a group of older women, $\frac{1}{3}$ of whom were noted to be obese, 50% were current or ex-smokers and 20% were suffering from high blood pressure, the results should come as no surprise. Even then the incidence of breast cancer, heart disease and stroke in the group receiving HRT increased by less than 1 in 1000 compared with the placebo group. If you can get your head around the statistics, for every 1000 women who took HRT the numbers of those who encountered any problems were hardly significant. As the media do they got hold of these results and made them sound sensational by referring to a 50% increase in diseases, which sounds quite frightening, whereas the actual number of women who developed breast cancer or heart disease was minimal.

It's a tragedy that this study, and the manner in which its results were presented, was allowed to influence the health choices of so many women in such an adverse fashion. Premarin and Provera, clearly not wise choices, are just two of the many forms of HRT available to women. What I employ in my practice is a different kind of HRT called bio-identical hormone replacement. This type of treatment utilises hormones which are derived from soy or wild yam, in a form which is more in line with individual needs. The major distinguishing factor here is the dosage and type of oestrogen and progesterone that is used. Oestrogen is the principal female hormone and there are three major forms of this hormone that are manufactured in the female body; oestradiol, oestrone and oestriol. Oestradiol and oestrone make up less than half of the total oestrogen complement but these are thought to be much more stimulating to breast tissue and therefore pose a greater threat. Oestriol, which comprises 80% of circulating oestrogen, is much less stimulating to the breast and possibly even protective. Conventional hormone replacement only incorporates oestradiol, which is also formulated from soy and wild yam whereas bio-identical therapy embraces all three oestrogens with oestriol occupying the lion's share of this formulation in doses that can be adjusted to suit hormone levels. The other core distinguishing feature is that regulation treatment involves the administration of progesterone, the other significant female hormone, in the form of a progestogen or Provera, which has a physical structure unlike that of progesterone. Remember I indicated earlier that Provera might share some of the responsibility for all the negative outcomes in the trials mentioned above. Like oestriol, progesterone in its true form is potentially much kinder to and protective of the female body. In the ensuing chapters you will discover how this kind of hormone replacement when combined with other hormones such as testosterone and DHEA can be used to manage female hormonal needs.

The fundamental question to be answered here is whether this type of treatment is safe and effective. Can this form of hormone replacement increase the risk of cancer or do we have a treatment that provides just the opposite, protection against the lethal demon that is the big C? Can bio-identical HRT turn you from an irritable, overweight grouch with little interest in sex who can't sleep at night because you are drenched in a lather of sweat into a healthy, happy and slim sexual athlete? Can this form of treatment also protect you against dreaded

Alzheimer's disease, prevent your bones from crumbling and protect your heart? This is what you are about to discover when you read this book.

What about vitamins? Do we need them or can we get enough of the essential nutrients that we need from the foods that we eat?   Some experts will tell you that there isn't any scientific evidence that vitamins and antioxidants can help to prevent the ageing process. (2) They claim that if you're looking to prevent heart disease and cancer then taking vitamins is a pointless exercise. What these experts are guilty of is examining the benefits of vitamins in isolation. They fail to recognise that combinations of vitamins rather than single nutrients do have protective effects. Vitamin C together with vitamin E has been associated with a decreased risk of death from cancer. The combination of zinc, selenium, vitamins C, E and beta-carotene has been found to boost the immune system and prevent respiratory tract infections. Zinc, copper, beta-carotene, vitamin C and vitamin E have been shown to delay the progression of age-related macular degeneration, the number one cause of blindness in the ageing population. No vitamin or antioxidant operates in nature on its own. Vitamins operate as a team and anyone who neglects to acknowledge this will not discover the true benefits of vitamin therapy. Repeatedly I find in my practice that my patients simply aren't getting enough of the essential vitamins that they need from the food they eat.   You only have to taste supermarket fruit and vegetables and compare these with fresh, organic produce to realise that these foods are devoid of essential nutrients. Although they may look reasonable they often taste waxy and bland and any resemblance they might have to the wholesome peach or apple they used to be is purely coincidental.

One thing is for sure there is virtually nothing that is more important than your health. Think what your life would be like if you suddenly contracted an illness which incapacitated you, making it impossible for you to carry out the simplest of daily functions or worse still you were struck down in your prime without any prior warning. If you take your health for granted this could happen to you.

Let me tell you about Jim, a gentleman in his late forties who came to see me complaining of chest pain that he had experienced the previous night. As the discomfort had gone away he was an unwilling visitor in my consulting rooms having been prodded into coming by his concerned wife, which is not an untypical scenario. I'm pleased to add that there are a growing number of men who are beginning to take a proactive interest in their health. Jim unfortunately wasn't very health conscious and hadn't had a checkup for a while. Aside from being slightly overweight, his blood pressure was normal, his heart sounded quite reasonable and his EKG, which measures the electrical current running through the heart and can be abnormal if a heart attack has been sustained, was also quite normal. Although I wasn't unduly worried, something in the back of my mind started to elicit gentle alarm bells so I thought it wise to send him to hospital for further tests.

I carried on with my daily activities and a few hours later I received a call from the doctor on-duty at the hospital who indicated that all the tests they had performed suggested that there was nothing wrong with Jim's heart and they were sending him home. A mere twenty minutes later the same doctor was on the line and in a most distraught fashion informed me that Jim was getting off the emergency room bed when he suddenly collapsed and went into a cardiac arrest. In simple terms this meant that his heart had stopped beating. All attempts at bringing Jim back to life failed and to the dismay and disbelief of the staff he was declared dead. You can imagine how difficult it was for me to return to my regular routine and I spent the rest of the day reflecting on this tragedy and the sometimes fragile nature of our existence.

Jim could be any one of us - a simple, hard-working, slightly overweight professional in his late forties who suddenly develops chest pain and dies 24 hours later. Jim's tragic circumstance and those of many others who are fatally struck down in the prime of their lives could have been prevented if only the right steps had been taken to avert these disasters. This is why it is so important to be pre-emptive about your health. So many of us, and this is probably human nature, only take action when things are going wrong. Sadly this may be the time when it is too late. It's like letting your motor vehicle, which most of us take in for an annual check-up, unlike our bodies, rust and rot and then expect the local service station to perform a miraculous resuscitation job. In truth we probably wouldn't let matters deteriorate to such an extent before we did something about it. If your car breaks down this might be mildly annoying and you might incur some financial hardship in order to replace the parts your vehicle needs. With your body you only get one shot. Once your body breaks down you might be in serious trouble and believe me you won't be able to drive into the repair shop and drive out the next day.

There is mounting evidence that all the diseases of ageing such as heart disease, dementia and cancer take many years to establish themselves in your body. Remarkably your blood vessels are thought to start blocking up somewhere between the age of five and ten. Alzheimer's dementia is thought to start in the twenties while cancer takes up to 40 years before it declares itself as a growth somewhere in your body. In other words your body can go downhill from a very early age and you won't even know about it until it's too late. Like Jim, in nearly 50% of cases, your first heart attack could be fatal and this would be the only indication that you had heart disease. In other words the sooner you take action the better. The converse is also true. There is always the potential to reshape your life and correct those circumstances that are impacting on your health in a negative fashion.

If you're dragging yourself through your working day, could fall asleep at the drop of a hat, notice that your memory is not what it used to be, have lost your sex drive and are finding it terribly difficult to lose weight and keep it off then reading this book will be extremely helpful to you. These are the kind of health concerns that I encounter regularly in my practice. Sadly these are also the kind of problems that conventional medicine struggles to fix. Have you presented to your doctor with similar complaints only to be told that there is nothing wrong with you once you have undergone the standard battery of blood tests and clinical investigations? What do you do then? What options are available to you and where do you turn? Well I've got good news for you. Help is at hand.

In this book you will discover how you can use hormones and vitamins to deal with the above-mentioned ailments and turn your health around. You will find out how you can boost your vitality utilising a programme that is tailored to your unique vitamin and hormone needs. You will also learn about specific tests that you can take to measure your vitamin and hormonal levels but even more importantly you will encounter a new set of investigations that will show you how your body is functioning at a cellular level. With the discovery of the genome, medicine is going to be heading down a completely different path. This is what Alvin Toffler, the renowned futurologist, foresaw in his book 'Future Shock' at least thirty years ago. He anticipated that science and technology would be utilised to individualise health care. By utilising genetic information doctors will be able to work out which hormones, vitamins and diet and even which medications can be accommodated to your specific genetic blueprint in order to optimise your health. This is medicine's future. Although conventional medical practice is falling behind a little, there are other doctors like myself who are already utilising the available technology to deliver this form of individualised medicine, which is the wave of the future. This is the fundamental difference between the wellness programme that I have been conducting at my clinic for the past four years and the traditional medical approach. Standard medical tests don't provide you with information as to how efficiently your cells are working. This is why you can often be told that you are normal and that there is nothing wrong when you know damn well that you are feeling awful.

In order for hormones and vitamins to do their job which to put it simply is to guide and energize your cells you simply have to ensure that all those tiny compartments where your life force is generated are functioning in the best possible fashion. Enter the revolutionary anti-ageing programme, which is designed to furnish you with a bird's eye view as to the workings of the cells of your body. If you often feel tired the investigations that are included in this programme should be able to tell you why and then equip you with those remedies that are designed to invigorate you. If poor memory, low sex drive and weight loss are your downfall then you should find the answers to these complex problems in this book.

You will also encounter novel approaches to common problems such as insomnia, depression and high blood pressure. How to boost your immune system, manage life-threatening illnesses such as HIV and multiple sclerosis as well as prevent and treat cancer, Parkinson's disease, Alzheimer's dementia and heart disease will be the substance of chapters to come. If wrinkles and hair loss are dampening your spirits then you might just be delivered from your funk.

This is also about the story of my life and the health challenges that I've had to negotiate on the long and winding road. I'll be sharing these with you as the tale unfolds.

CHAPTER 3

From Fatigue to Energy

Many of us spend so much of our day pushing ourselves, looking after the children, racing to get to work, rushing to our next appointment, getting home late, eating on the run, cramming as much as we can into a day that just doesn't appear to provide us with all the time we need. We always seem to be behind the eight ball, fighting desperately to keep pace with our torrid existence, struggling to stay afloat. Is it any wonder that many of us become exhausted and spent? I don't encounter that many people who are brimming with energy and vigour and yet are calm and peaceful. Those who have found their power, their passion and their purpose and are experiencing limitless flowing energy are few and far between.

The opposite is the grim reality for most. Fatigue can be one of the most debilitating health problems that you can experience. If you don't have energy you simply can't function. There's nothing worse than starting your day with virtually no energy because all your resources are depleted and forcing yourself through the day without any vitality. Have you ever found yourself dying to fall asleep after lunch or nearly nodding off when you're behind the wheel of your car driving to your next appointment? If this is an ongoing problem then you need to read on, as there's probably something very correctable about this debilitating and somewhat scary state of affairs. The most extreme form of this ailment is chronic fatigue syndrome that can be so overwhelming as to prevent you from even getting out of bed or having a shower.   How do you deal with exhaustion once the conventional medical tests have ruled out iron deficiency, glandular fever or any other medical illness? Can hormones and vitamins provide the answers? Can these critical chemicals help to make you ready for the day when you will discover your power?   Can they provide you with the energy and vitality that you are lacking before accessing the power takes you to the next level?

As we age it seems to become that much harder to execute those daily functions that we take for granted. Instead we are faced with diminishing energy, reduced mental capacity, an expanding waistline and the inexorable power of nature and gravity leading to all those wrinkles, sags and bulges that appear to be the depressingly inevitable consequence of ageing. Fascinatingly a lot of what happens around the ageing process hinges on three basic operations. Firstly our cells need to be provided with oxygen and water. These are the most vital nutrients. Starve your cells of oxygen for more than five minutes and they will die. So much of the air we breathe is unclean and polluted and because of our stressful lives many of us have lost the capacity to breathe deeply. Instead we are driven by shallow breathing which compromises our energy. A full in-breath should commence from your belly button. From there the movement should radiate upwards allowing your upper chest to expand so that you get the maximal entry of air into your lungs.

Try doing this now.   Place your hand over your lower abdomen and as your breathe in allow your body to gently push your hand away.   Then take the air into your lungs and notice how the upper part of your chest moves upwards and appears to enlarge.   Do this for five breaths and notice how it feels. The practice of yoga is one way to discover the lost art of effective breathing. Inhaling and exhaling in the proper fashion forms the basis of good yoga practice and doing this kind of activity regularly can help to establish the deep, enlivening breath that eludes many of us.

Another way to ensure that you breathe good quality air is to install an air humidifier in your home. This will remove some of the contaminants that pollute your home environment. If we cannot survive without oxygen then water would have to be the next most critical nutrient. Human beings can live without food for thirty to forty days but without water we would perish within five. We are comprised of 70% water and our cells remain fluid and functional because of this life-giving substance. Thirst is not a good way to sense that you are getting enough water as your cells become dehydrated long before you experience the need to drink. As a general rule consuming 5-6 glasses per day is considered to be sufficient with filtered water being the best way to obtain this essential substance. The best water filter would be the one the removes all the contaminants that pollute your water supply. Reverse osmosis and ceramic filtration systems are considered to be the most effective for doing this.

Secondly how efficiently we use sugar or glucose to generate energy is crucial. Our bodies consist of millions of tiny cells, which need energy to survive and function. This energy comes from glucose and as long as this basic activity proceeds in an orderly fashion all is well. What we need to do is get the glucose into our cells and once it's there use it in a businesslike way to provide energy. Once this system starts to break down then the characteristic features of ageing can start to take hold. Thirdly we need to deal successfully with the accumulation of free radicals. These are chemicals that have the power to destroy us. If our cells are exposed to an excess of free radicals they will be overwhelmed. As we get older we tend to accumulate free radicals and our ability to defend ourselves diminishes. The good news is that this is not universally true. There are a group of individuals who appear to have found the magic solution to the metabolic difficulties that we have to deal with, as we get older. A recent study has shown that healthy centenarians have less free radical stress and efficient glucose metabolism. (1) In other words if you want to stay around for as long as possible and you want to remain in the best shape make sure that your glucose is working for you and you have the capacity to deal effectively with free radicals. Naturally what you want to know is how you can achieve this. Hormones and vitamins are the essential ingredients that make it easy for our cells to utilise glucose to generate energy. They also help to protect us against free radicals. Once you understand how these operate then you can take the appropriate action to ensure that your cells have all the hormones and vitamins they need. Let's firstly take a look at the various hormones and how they work.

GROWTH HORMONE

This hormone is considered to be the superman of all hormones as far as anti-ageing benefits are concerned. Ask any anti-ageing specialist and they will tell you that this hormone has the ability to boost your energy, make you lose weight, improve your physique, rejuvenate your skin and invigorate your mind. In fact, renowned Belgian Endocrinologist and anti-ageing specialist Thierry Hertoghe goes so far as to say that if you have all those external signs of ageing such as thinning hair, sagging cheeks and a flabby belly combined with irritability, anxiety and exhaustion, then it is highly likely that you are deficient in growth hormone and replacing this hormone will turn all these symptoms around. There is the notion that you grow old because your body does not produce enough growth hormone. If you want to preserve your muscles, prevent weight gain and maintain a good quality of life with ample energy then what you have to do is restore flagging growth hormone levels. Elite athletes are renowned for taking growth hormone as it makes them recover more quickly and boosts their muscle growth.

As the name suggests growth hormone is responsible for making our bones and muscles grow. This hormone helps us to maintain good body composition and has the potential to make us function more effectively both in body and in mind. There is another hormone associated with growth hormone called IGF-1 that is predominantly produced by the liver. IGF-1 is thought to be growth hormone's partner as it performs a similar function.

If your growth hormone levels are low and you are suffering from excessive fatigue, weakness, depression and a potbelly that doesn't want to go away then boosting your levels of this hormone might help to renew your energy and deal effectively with these debilitating problems. How do you know if your hormone levels are low? One of the ways to establish this is to have your IGF-1 levels measured which is an indirect way of assessing how much growth hormone your body is producing. Unfortunately you can't measure your growth hormone levels directly via a blood test as your body produces very little growth hormone during the day. Growth hormone is manufactured predominantly at night when you sleep which is why it's important to get a good night's rest. Low thyroid hormone, imperfect liver function and the presence of excessive levels of oestrogen can reduce IGF-1 and are the factors that need to be recognized when you have this test.

The normal range for IGF-1 is 9-38nmol/Litre. An optimal level for IGF-1 would be 25-30nmol/Litre and I usually initiate treatment when this level is around 20 or below. There are many different strategies that you can adopt to increase growth hormone.

Increasing growth hormone:

- Exercise regularly and include weight training at least three times a week for half-an hour. Increasing your weights on a regular basis is also a good idea. Lessening the amount of repetitions you do while using heavier weights would improve your muscle mass and intensify growth hormone stimulation. If you can, incorporate high intensity exercise such as sprinting and squash.
- Losing weight and eating less would be beneficial. Reducing your food consumption can be a real challenge. For those of you who are horrified by this concept stay tuned as I have some novel ideas later in the book as to how you can achieve similar results by using a certain antioxidant without altering your dietary habits.
- Optimise your levels of testosterone, thyroid hormone, melatonin and DHEA. These hormones increase growth hormone production and will be discussed shortly.
- Introducing growth hormone promoting agents is nice way to encourage the body to produce more growth hormone. This method leads to far fewer side-effects and allows your body to decide when enough is enough. Typically these promoting agents are amino acids, which are the building blocks for proteins. For example, taking 6 grams a day of L-arginine would stimulate growth hormone production. You can combine amino acids to achieve a similar result. Another option would be to take 2 grams of L-arginine together with 1 gram

of L-ornithine or 1500mg of L-arginine with 1500mg of L-lysine. There is another study, which shows that combining 2½ grams of glutamine with the same amount of glycine and adding 1 gram of the B vitamin niacin can increase growth hormone levels. I have developed an affinity for the product trans-D tropin, which includes a number of amino acids and other nutrients designed to stimulate growth hormone formation. This product can be obtained from a company called College Pharmacy in the USA. My patients like this formulation as it helps to boost muscle mass and increase energy especially when applied just before a workout. A healthy dose is 15 drops applied to your forearm once - twice daily 5 days a week with a rest on the weekend.

- Obviously the most profound way to raise your exposure to growth hormone is via injections of this substance using a very small needle just under your skin. You'll be pleased to know the injection is almost painless and you should start off with ¼ -½ of an international unit taken each day from Monday to Friday either in the morning or evening. Some say the evening is better as your cells are more receptive at this time while others claim that morning injections would be the preferred option as this would provide you with the benefits of growth hormone at a time when your body is producing very little. It's a good idea to give your cells a rest on the weekend, as you don't want your receptors to be flooded with too much hormonal stimulation. This allows your receptors time to recuperate so that your cells remain receptive and ready. Because you are exposing yourself to a stronger form of hormone treatment you also have to watch out for all the side-effects including fluid retention, joint and muscle pain and headaches. This is why it's important to start off with a low dose and have your IGF-1 levels monitored regularly. With the normal range for IGF-1 being 11-36nmol/Litre, I like to bring the IGF-1 level into a zone, which I believe to be the most beneficial, this being around the 20-29nmol/litre mark.

Be Careful when you ignite your engine with rocket fuel

This is the point with growth hormone replacement. Igniting your engine with rocket fuel is going to lead to some wear and tear along the way. Supercharging your cells will lead to the accumulation of more free radicals. This is when you need to fortify yourself with extra antioxidants to minimise any adverse events while maximising your benefits. Once you commence this treatment or any form of hormone replacement for that matter you need to be eternally vigilant. This means that men need to have regular prostate checks by means of blood tests and internal investigations, while periodic mammograms and gynaecological surveillance is my recommendation for women. There are studies which demonstrate a connection between high growth hormone as well as elevated IGF-1 levels and various cancers including breast, prostate and bowel cancer. This is why you have to be careful and ensure that your IGF-1 levels don't increase excessively. In the chapter on cancer prevention you will discover how you can protect yourself as much as is humanly possible against the development of various cancers.

TESTOSTERONE

Testosterone is the major male hormone. In a nutshell it's what makes a man a man.

If your levels of this hormone are low then boosting testosterone can increase your energy and provide you with a number of benefits. In 2003 a comprehensive review in the Journal of the American Geriatric Society collated all those studies from January 1966 till the end of October 2001, which explored testosterone supplementation in males over the age of 45 who were low in testosterone. (2)

Here were the most prominent findings:

- Testosterone supplementation improved energy, well-being and alleviated depression.
- Almost universally the men became leaner and thinner. They lost fat and gained muscle.
- In some trials improvements in memory were noted.
- Bones became less brittle as was evidenced by improved bone mineral density, which is a

very important finding. Men suffer from
osteoporosis almost as much as women.

- Libido, which is sexual desire, was enhanced
  and in some cases the quality of their erections
  improved especially when testosterone levels
  were really low.
- Men with heart disease experienced
  improvements in their condition. They were
  able to exercise more without discomfort.
  LDL, the bad cholesterol, was reduced with no
  change in HDL, the good cholesterol.
- Minimal changes in prostate specific antigen
  (PSA) were noted. The PSA is the blood test
  which evaluates prostate status. It's not a
  definitive estimation of prostate cancer as
  there isn't such a test but once this measure
  starts to go up then the prostate needs specialist
  attention.

In summary the authors of this article suggest that
'testosterone replacement in mildly androgen-deficient older
men (older being from the age of 45 onwards which is a little
harsh) may have potentially beneficial effects on body
composition, muscle strength, sexual functioning, subjective
well-being and manifestations of heart disease.' The normal
range for testosterone is 8-38nmol/Litre. In these studies men
received testosterone if their levels were anywhere between 8-
15nmol/Litre and the aim of the treatment was to restore their
levels to between 15-20nmol/Litre.

If you have low testosterone levels, which would be
below 15nmol/Litre and you are suffering from any of the

following problems then enhancing your levels of this hormone might lead to a number of benefits:

> ## Features of low testosterone
>
> - Fatigue, irritability, depression and diminished mental capacity.
> - Lessening of sexual desire with reduced erectile potency and absence of nocturnal erections.
> - Decrease in muscle mass with associated loss of strength.
> - Increase in fat mass.
> - Decrease in bone density.
> - Decrease in body hair with thinning of skin and the development of wrinkles.

If you have a number of these difficulties then your benefits might be far more tangible. When you have your testosterone levels measured there is another molecule, which is assessed, called sex hormone binding globulin. This is a carrier protein, which has the job of transporting testosterone around the body to those places where this hormone does its thing. The trouble is that sex hormone binding globulin likes holding on to testosterone and the older you get the more your body produces this protein which leads to a firmer grip on the hormone in question. Sex hormone binding globulin also goes up if your liver isn't working too well or if you are exposed to excessive amounts of thyroid hormone or oestrogen, the female hormone, which is also manufactured in the male body in lesser amounts. Oestrogen increases though, once you start to put on weight. Your testosterone levels might be reasonable but if your sex hormone globulin is high then the potency of this hormone will be reduced. This is why you need to ensure that you stay in shape and treat your liver with the utmost respect. If this means cutting back on alcohol consumption then so be it. Getting your doctor to check your thyroid hormone levels, especially if your body is producing too much sex hormone binding globulin, would also be important.

If your testosterone levels are low and you don't have much energy together with some of the other characteristics of androgen deficiency what steps can you take to bolster your supply of this hormone?

Boosting testosterone

- Make sure that you consume adequate amounts of protein. If you weigh 85kg your diet should be comprised of 70-90grams of protein daily. For example, the average piece of steak would make up approximately 15grams of protein, one egg would equal 10grams of protein. Vegetarians might struggle here as their diets can be lacking in protein. I always advise vegetarians to take protein supplements in the form of a powder made from soy or rice protein, which can be blended with fruit and soy or rice milk to make a delicious smoothie. This is a very enjoyable way of obtaining at least 30 extra grams of protein.

- Zinc supplementation has the ability to increase testosterone levels. This is especially true if you are zinc deficient. One way to assess whether this is the case is to have what is called a zinc taste test, which is a very simple way to determine your zinc status. As this mineral affects your sense of taste you will not do well on this test if your zinc levels are low. Taking 30mg of zinc daily should have some impact on your testosterone status.

- Regular exercise boosts testosterone as does rooting for (supporting) the winning team. (no pun intended) Exercise helps to reduce stress which also goes some way to preserving the good old male hormone.

- Maintaining your optimal weight is beneficial. If you are overweight your body will make extra amounts of the female hormone oestrogen, which will lead to lower testosterone levels.

- Looking after your liver is a must. If this organ isn't working well oestrogen will accumulate and that's not good news for testosterone. Resisting the temptation to have that extra glass of wine or bottle of beer would be prudent. Drinking more than two cups of coffee a day and wearing tight underwear also increase oestrogen.

- There is some evidence that taking the herb tribulus terrestris will increase testosterone. You have to see to it that you take 250mg of the active component of the herb three times daily.

- The hormones DHEA and androstenediol both have the potential to raise testosterone levels. The latter has been used by athletes for this purpose. However both of these hormones also have the ability to stimulate oestrogen production, which is the very hormone that the male body doesn't want too much of. Both sexes need each other's hormones but they need to coexist in the right proportions. Although most of the scientific literature indicates that DHEA makes testosterone in the female body, but has a greater tendency to promote the production of oestrogen in men, I don't usually find this to be the case especially when weight is maintained within the ideal range.

- Although it would be nice to encourage your body to produce more testosterone this method does not always prove to be the most effective. Naturally the most powerful way to augment testosterone is to take the hormone itself. I have found that the best way to administer testosterone is via a cream or troche, which is a lozenge that is placed inside the cheek or under the tongue. These formulations are put together by compounding pharmacies and they are tailor-made to a doctor's prescription which is the beauty of this approach, as one size does not fit all. Wild yam or soy are the sources from which these hormones are derived. With regard to the cream the starting dose is 25-50 mg applied to the forearm or the angle of the jaw once to twice daily. Troches are usually commenced at a similar dose. The normal male range for testosterone is 8-38nmol/Litre and the aim of this treatment is to elevate testosterone levels to anywhere between 18-25nmol/Litre. I have had patients as young as their late thirties all the way up to the mature age of 75 who have benefited from taking testosterone to alleviate their fatigue and improve their sexual energy.

With regard to testosterone therapy you need to have your hormonal levels monitored every 3-6 months to make sure that they remain within an acceptable range. Along with testosterone you should also have your dihydrotestosterone (DHT) and oestrogen levels measured. DHT is the stronger form of the male hormone that is made from testosterone via an enzyme called 5 alpha reductase. Although we have yet to discover what makes the prostate enlarge or develop cancer there is limited evidence that having too much DHT could pose some problems for the prostate. Equally, excessive amounts of oestrogen, which is manufactured from testosterone via an enzyme called aromatase, could be bad news for the prostate. More about this in the cancer chapter. It is vital that you have your PSA measured via a blood test when you have your hormones evaluated. Together with a digital examination of your prostate which should be done annually from the age of fifty, the PSA gives you some indication of your prostate status. If your PSA starts to climb, you need to involve your friendly urologist, a specialist who deals with disorders of the prostate.

As testosterone has the ability to increase your red cell and haemoglobin levels you should also have your blood count checked periodically. You need to prevent these levels from escalating as this would lead to your blood becoming too thick and sludgy. At the same time you should have your cholesterol levels monitored along with HDL and LDL, the good and bad cholesterol, to ensure that these remain within healthy parameters.

So much for testosterone for men but what about this hormone for women? Would testosterone benefit female energy?

TESTOSTERONE FOR WOMEN

Just to show that men aren't about to steal all the menopause thunder, women have coined their own syndrome which describes the decline in female testosterone with age. Yes, women also have to endure male menopause if you follow my meaning. This is because the female body produces testosterone albeit in much lesser amounts than the male. Between the age of 20 and 45 there is a substantial decline in the production of this hormone so that some women may actually suffer from a disorder that has neatly been termed the 'female androgen insufficiency syndrome.'

Low testosterone in women

- Persistent fatigue
- Low libido with a decrease in sexual desire and fantasy
- Diminished sense of well-being
- Thinning or loss of pubic hair
- Decreased muscle mass
- Weakening of bone strength termed osteopenia leading to osteoporosis
- Total testosterone being below the lower quartile of the normal range

The final point is the crucial one. If your testosterone is low, as evidenced by a blood test, and you qualify with other features of this syndrome then you may well benefit from testosterone supplementation. As the normal range for women is 1-4.5nmol/Litre, you should look at treatment if your levels are less than 2nmol/Litre. The aim is to bring your testosterone to around 3nmol/Litre. If you are worried about developing masculine features this shouldn't happen if your testosterone is maintained at this healthy level. Any development of excess body hair or any other signs of maleness are totally reversible once your dose of testosterone is reduced or terminated if you are unhappy with the results. In the menopause chapter I will discuss how I implement this treatment and how it is monitored as I administer testosterone in conjunction with a number of other hormones.

Is testosterone safe for women? There are an abundance of studies investigating the relationship between testosterone and breast cancer. While some studies suggest that testosterone might be protective there are also those that show that having too much testosterone or the other female hormones can be detrimental. In other words just as men need the right amount of testosterone similar principles apply to women. Enough is as good as a feast and too much could lead to adverse outcomes.

OESTROGEN

Oestrogen is to the female as testosterone is to the male. This hormone defines the essence of femininity. The growth and development of the vagina, the enlargement of the breasts and the formation of the mature female body are due to the presence of oestrogen. This hormone is responsible for looking after every cell and function in the female body. From the depths of your heart to the inner recesses of your brain, the fine lines of your skin to the firm lines of your body, the blooming of your sexuality to the source of your female energy, it all hinges on the presence of oestrogen. On average women live 10 years longer than men. This might result from the awesome power of oestrogen as this hormone has the ability to significantly enhance the body's antioxidant defensive capacities, to protect against heart disease and to boost the immune system.

**Here is a list of the symptoms that result
from oestrogen deficiency:**

- Hot flushes
- Vaginal dryness
- Crawling sensations under the skin
- Wrinkles, dry skin and poor skin texture
- Poor memory
- Lack of sexual desire
- Depression
- Hair loss with male distribution of body hair on the face
- Bladder infections
- Lack of energy
- Dry eyes
- Menstrual headaches
- Irregular periods
- Cessation of periods
- Insomnia
- Osteoporosis
- Night sweats

If you suspect that you are low in oestrogen then you need to have your hormone levels measured. The best time to do this is one week before your period, which is also an ideal time to assess progesterone production, the other major female hormone. While oestrogen will not supercharge you with energy it will provide you with a more sustainable form of vitality and it will make you feel better and alleviate many of these symptoms. Oestrogen is a replenishing, nurturing hormone and there is some evidence that it helps glucose to enter your cells, which is vital for energy production. Once you start taking oestrogen you need to make sure that you don't experience the excesses of this hormone.

Excess oestrogen can lead to:

- Anxiety
- Irritability
- Nervous tension
- Swollen breasts and breast cysts
- Fluid retention
- Weight gain (possibly)
- Sugar cravings

If you are experiencing these symptoms you need to reduce your dose. Excess oestrogen also gets in the way of thyroid hormone function and as you will discover it is really important for your energy levels that your thyroid performs unchecked by any negative hormonal influences. Aside from your dose of hormones being too high oestrogen needs to be processed and eliminated by your gut and your liver meaning that you have to keep these two organs in good shape.

PROGESTERONE

This hormone is produced in the second half of your menstrual cycle with oestrogen dominating the first half. While oestrogen is responsible for building the lining of the uterus during the initial part of the menstrual cycle, progesterone has to ensure that this lining is maintained so that any fertilised egg has a ready made home in which it can nestle and grow.

> **Insufficient progesterone can result in:**
>
> - Anxiety
> - Irritability
> - Premenstrual headaches
> - Painful, swollen breasts
> - Heavy periods with lots of discomfort
> - Restless sleep

Having too much progesterone, usually due to overdosing, is also counterproductive as this hormone has the ability to impede the entry of glucose into your cells, which will compromise your energy. Excesses can also lead to sleepiness, weight gain and depression.

If you're struggling to get a good nights rest taking a small amount of this hormone before you go to sleep may be just the tonic you need to cure your insomnia.

THYROID HORMONE

This hormone has a substantial impact on your well-being. Glucose and energy become readily available once your thyroid hormone is happily pulsing around your body. If you aren't manufacturing enough of this hormone everything tends to slow down. You become tired, mentally sluggish, constipated and your circulation is compromised. Thyroid hormone sees to it that all the organs and cells of your body receive all the nutrients they need in a timely and efficient fashion. Imagine how hungry and frustrated you'd become if you ordered room service and three hours later you were still waiting for your meal. This is how your body struggles if your thyroid hormone fails to deliver.

Features of low thyroid hormone

- Fatigue which is worse in the morning and may improve as the day progresses
- Cold hands and feet
- Weight gain
- Fluid retention
- Depression
- Mental dullness
- Impaired concentration
- Hair loss
- Dry eyes
- Dry and rough skin
- Headaches
- Low libido
- Puffy face
- Elevated cholesterol
- Nocturnal cramps
- Carpal tunnel syndrome
- Irritability
- Anxiety and panic attacks

Low thyroid function can weaken your immune system, accelerate heart disease and is even associated with Alzheimer's dementia.

There are a number of factors that lower your thyroid hormone levels:

- High stress levels with elevated cortisol and low DHEA
- Fasting
- Low selenium levels
- Low zinc status
- Low vitamin B12 levels
- Low melatonin
- Low growth hormone
- Low progesterone
- High oestrogen
- Insufficient iodine
- Excessive exposure to the heavy metals lead and cadmium
- Autoimmune thyroid disease which increases with ageing

Your thyroid gland requires the right blend of hormones and nutrients to thrive. A staggering 10% of the adult population of the USA suffer from the effects of low thyroid function with women occupying a lion's share of this statistic. If you suspect that you have insufficient thyroid hormone as evidenced by a mix of the symptoms mentioned above then you need to have your thyroid hormones measured. This is when matters become interesting, as the conventional medical approach will fail you as it sometimes does. There are two principal thyroid hormones, which are produced by the thyroid gland; thyroxine also known as T4 and triiodothyronine or T3. Thyroid-stimulating hormone (TSH), produced in the pituitary gland, has the job of encouraging your thyroid gland to manufacture T4 and T3. When your thyroid gland fails to uphold its end of the bargain then the pituitary will increase TSH in order to step up the production of T4 and T3. The normal range of TSH is 0.30-4.00mIU/Litre and in order to determine whether you have enough thyroid hormones your doctor will usually measure only TSH. If this hormone lies within acceptable limits there is no need to quantify T4 and T3 and, according to established medical wisdom, you don't have a problem. Unfortunately this argument has its limitations, as the range of TSH is far too broad. Your T4 and T3 might reside at the lower limit of their range which is 2.5-6.0pmol/Litre for T3 and 10-25pmol/Litre for T4 and this will not be reflected in your TSH evaluation. Your body has to convert T4 to T3, which is the far more potent of the two hormones and the success of this process hardly impacts your TSH levels. Incidentally this process takes place predominantly in your liver. There is another hormone called reverse T3 (RT3) which blocks the activity of T3 and increases when you are stressed or you decide to fast or you are zinc or selenium deficient. Once again your TSH will be untouched when this happens. Finally there is a disorder called 'sick euthyroid syndrome' which indicates that your thyroid function is ostensibly normal yet you are suffering from the effects of a troubled thyroid. In this scenario your T4 is normal, your T3 is low and your TSH lies within range.

In other words there is more than sufficient evidence to support the notion that simply quantifying TSH is hardly an adequate reflection of the totality of your thyroid hormone activity. You really should have your T4, T3 and RT3 estimated to get the full picture. Some suggest that you take your temperature first thing in the morning over a sequence of days to get a sense of what is happening in your cells. It's all very well having sufficient quantities of thyroid hormones in your bloodstream but you need these hormones to activate your cells in the appropriate manner to obtain a proper evaluation of your thyroid function. If your temperature is constantly below 36.5° C then it is highly likely that you are experiencing the effects of low thyroid activity.

MANAGING LOW THYROID FUNCTION

Your thyroid function is a perfect barometer of hormonal and cellular harmony. If your hormones are in balance, the right nutrients are present, and your cells are receptive and ready then you shouldn't experience any of the effects of low thyroid function. However if you do have symptoms then it would be a good idea to address all the contributing factors mentioned above if you want to enjoy the benefits of a fully operational thyroid. Regrettably this is not what usually happens when you consult with your average doctor. Mostly you will commence treatment with thyroxine once it is established that your thyroid function is low. That this band-aid type of approach sometimes does the trick is a miracle. In my practice I see patients who have not benefited from this treatment and this is when it becomes important to investigate all those factors that impair thyroid function. Once you've corrected your imbalances there are other options for thyroid hormone treatment.

ARMOUR THYROID

This is a desiccated thyroid extract of porcine origin containing both T4 and T3. Routine treatment with thyroxine consisting only of T4 doesn't ensure that you are provided with the more powerful thyroid hormone, which is T3. This is why this treatment sometimes fails. A study has shown that combination treatments of T4 and T3 are superior to solitary T4 for boosting mood and mental function. (3) You need to commence at 15mg daily and you can increase your dose on a weekly basis to 60mg daily or even more if your symptoms have not abated. If you're not too keen on receiving hormones that are made from pig thyroid, which is understandable, then a compounding pharmacy can also dispense sustained release physiologic thyroid hormone extract. A dose, which combines 11.2mcg of T4 and 3.4mcg of T3, would approximate 15mg of Armour thyroid.

As you would with any hormone treatment, you need to have your hormonal levels monitored by your doctor. When you start this therapy it is important that you make sure that your adrenals are fully operational. This can be done by measuring your adrenal hormones including DHEA and cortisol, which I'll be discussing shortly. If you commence this treatment and you don't have enough of these hormones then taking too much Armour thyroid can make you feel unwell and you might need to reduce your dose. Armour thyroid can be taken indefinitely.

TRIIODOTHYRONINE AND SLOW RELEASE T3

Another alternative is to take T3 on its own. My preference is to use the slow release formulation. This needs to be initiated at a very low dose of 15mcg twice daily and can be increased depending upon your response to this therapy including the increase in temperature and your hormone levels. As mentioned earlier your adrenals should be working well when you start slow release T3.

CORTISOL

Your thyroid exerts metabolic control but your adrenal glands are just as important as they have the responsibility to produce those hormones that get you out of bed in the morning and sustain you as the day progresses. In fact cortisol and thyroid hormone depend upon each other for optimal function. You need thyroid hormone to manufacture cortisol and your body has to provide you with just the right amount of cortisol to get the best out of thyroid hormone. Cortisol is the hormone that jumpstarts your day as its production peaks in the early morning and then goes down during the day.

When you are low in cortisol you may experience the following:

- Light-headedness especially when standing due to low blood pressure
- Early morning fatigue
- Weakness
- Irritability
- Sugar cravings
- Increased skin pigmentation

If you want to prod your adrenals into generating more cortisol then you have to look to herbal remedies such as ginseng, withania and liquorice. Your adrenals also need the amino acid tyrosine, vitamins C, E and the B complex together with the minerals zinc and magnesium to achieve their best function.

The thing about cortisol is that you want the right amount of this hormone as too much can reduce your energy, compromise your immune system, increase your weight and weaken your bones. As you get older your levels of this hormone tend to overstay their welcome in your system and this is one of the factors that is thought to hasten the ageing process. There is a neat little supplement called phosphatidylserine that can reign in your cortisol if your body is producing excessive amounts of this hormone. One of the ways to discover whether your body is outlaying too much cortisol is to have your hormone levels measured via a blood test, which should be performed first thing in the morning and then in the early afternoon. The normal range for morning cortisol is 138-650nmol/Litre, while that for the afternoon assay is 70-325nmol/Litre.

DHEA

This is quite a fascinating hormone as we have yet to determine all that it does in the body. One of its major roles is that of a prohormone or a wellspring for the formation of other hormones. With regard to women it is the primary source of female and male hormones after the menopause and even before this transition DHEA contributes to the formation of testosterone and oestrogen. As far is the male is concerned DHEA is the progenitor of testosterone but this contribution appears to be less significant than in the female experience.

The presence of this hormone is ubiquitous as there's hardly an organ in the body that doesn't benefit from the existence of DHEA.

Low DHEA is associated with:

- Fatigue
- Pre-menopausal breast and ovarian cancer
- Lupus
- Rheumatoid arthritis
- Multiple sclerosis
- Impaired immunity
- Heart disease
- Erectile dysfunction
- Diminished libido in women
- Memory loss
- Alzheimer's disease
- Decreased well-being
- Depression
- Increased mortality in men

As meditation increases DHEA this hormone can be viewed as having a calming effect on the body. You could say it generates the energy of the marathon runner. We're talking endurance rather than performance. DHEA moderates the overzealousness of cortisol thereby allowing you to stay around for the long haul.

So there we have it. All the primary hormones that combine in a highly ordered and mutually dependent fashion to choreograph the cellular dance of our daily lives. If you are feeling drained then a good place to start would be to have all your hormone levels measured and if any of these are low then you need to take the necessary steps to renew declining hormone levels. Is it wise to replace these powerful chemicals once we age and our bodies start to shut down? Is the decline in hormones with ageing nature's way of protecting us against the development of cancer? You could argue for and against this proposition but until all the scientific evidence is available I'm going to stick my neck out and say that if you want to experience maximal energy then opting to re-ignite flagging hormone levels would appear to be the way forward. Now let's see how vitamins fit into the scheme of things.

Vitamins help you to dance

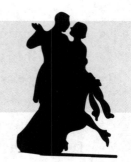

VITAMINS

If hormones orchestrate your cells then vitamins and minerals are the players that produce the sweet music which shapes your daily dance. While hormones drive your cells, vitamins and minerals facilitate the many biochemical reactions that generate the energy without which you would not be able to function. Deficiencies of these essential nutrients dampen your spirits, dull your intellect, and in extreme cases lead to disease states such as scurvy, beri-beri and rickets, which are typical of severe vitamin insufficiency. The trouble is that these diseases are virtually unheard of in most western societies. Almost no-one suffers from a profound lack of any essential nutrients. Does this mean that we are getting all the vitamins we need and that supplements are an expensive waste of time?

Until recently this was the conventional wisdom. A varied diet high in vegetables, fruits and grains was thought to be all that you needed to guarantee a healthy life. Back in 1993 a thirteen-year study on no fewer than 10,578 Americans conducted by a research team from the Centre for Disease Control and Prevention in Atlanta declared to the world that there was no evidence of increased longevity among vitamin and mineral supplement users. (4) Then along came a review reported in no less a publication than the highly prestigious Journal of the American Medical Association, which boldly suggested that we all need vitamin supplements. (5) This article indicated that we need extra folic acid and B vitamins to protect against heart disease, breast and bowel cancer, while increased vitamin E and lycopene found in tomatoes were shown to reduce the risk of prostate cancer.

In fact there are many more reasons for turning to these vital chemicals. Storing food in the refrigerator and then heating it, eating on the run, alcohol consumption, stress, junk foods, poor absorption and ageing precludes diet alone from providing an optimal supply of vitamins.

How do you know whether you are lacking in vitamins? There are a whole host of easily identifiable clues. Certainly if you're fatigued and you are suffering from any of the following including depression, dermatitis, anxiety, shortness of breath, burning feet, a red tongue, poor memory, irritability and sores at the side of your mouth that don't heal, chances are that you are suffering from a deficiency of the B group vitamins. Unfortunately blood tests that investigate your vitamin status won't always tell you how effectively your vitamins are functioning in your cells. I use an ingenious method of investigation devised by a very astute Brisbane physician who constructed a questionnaire, which focuses on the above symptoms and others resulting from vitamin deficiencies. Responses to these questions generate a graph, which identifies a wide spectrum of nutrient deficiencies including all the vitamins and essential minerals. I have incorporated this questionnaire in my wellness programme for quite a while now and have found that a large majority of my patients eke out their daily existence suffering from the lack of a whole range of nutrients.

These are the vitamins, minerals and antioxidants that I prescribe most often to boost energy:

- The B vitamin complex 100mg of each vitamin
- Vitamin C 2000mg in divided doses
- Vitamin E 400i.u. comprising mixed tocopherols and 50mg tocotrienols
- Magnesium diglycinate 500mg
- Zinc sulphate 30mg
- Coenzyme Q10 100mg
- Acetyl-L-carnitine 1000mg
- Alpha-lipoic acid 200mg

The above is a daily regimen, which should be taken in the morning after breakfast. Naturally this recipe has to be tailored to individual needs. The B complex vitamins are very good stress-busters while vitamin C fuels adrenal function. Zinc and magnesium are essential for cellular energy. Coenzyme Q10 and alpha-lipoic acid are powerful antioxidants that help your mitochondria or your cellular batteries to function more efficiently. Acetyl-L-carnitine, an amino acid complex which assists with fat metabolism, provides your mitochondria with a ready source of energy. Vitamin E is a complex antioxidant that we'll visit in more detail when we explore ways to look after your heart and your brain.

One of the most important components of your well-being is a healthy bowel. Naturopathic physicians claim that if your bowel is right the rest of you follows suit so let's outline the essential features of a robust digestive process.

A HEALTHY BOWEL

If you want to derive the full benefit from all those nutritious foods that you are sending the way of your digestive tract as well as the supplements you are taking then you have to ensure that you're digesting and absorbing what you put in your mouth. It's very easy to tell whether your digestive system is in good working order. Firstly, you should be relatively free of those symptoms which indicate that your bowels simply aren't functioning properly. Excessive burping, bloating and flatulence, which don't exactly endear you to your intimates, are pointers to an unhealthy bowel. This means that either you are eating those foods which don't agree with you or you are not producing enough of those digestive juices which are responsible for breaking down the food you eat into small particles that can be absorbed by your digestive tract. Secondly you should be moving your bowels every day and your stools should be brown, formed and they should float. Far be it from me to make every one of you obsessive stool watchers but let's face it, most of us love our bowel motions, so why not pay that extra attention to the health of your bowel? If you are one of the many who are unhappy with the performance of your digestive tract here's what you can do.

OPTIMISING BOWEL HEALTH

1.   Find out if you have food allergies/intolerance. This can be difficult as you may not be allergic to specific foods in the classical sense but you may have reactions that are more subtle leading to such symptoms as fatigue, headaches, fuzzy headedness, acne, eczema, psoriasis and sinus congestion. Bad breath and a white coating on your tongue are further indications that something in your diet might not be agreeing with you. Your tongue should have a smooth pink appearance. Have a look at your tongue in the mirror right now. If your tongue is covered with a white film chances are that you are eating something that your body doesn't like or you are not digesting your food adequately. Another way that you can tell whether you are eating the wrong foods or have a digestive imbalance is to ask those who are close to you about your breath. Bad breath is a classic symptom of poor digestive health.

In my practice I start off with the conventional skin prick tests and I also perform a blood test investigating gliadin and candida antibodies. Gliadin antibodies cover the gluten containing range of foods found in wheat, rye, oats and barley. If anyone has elevated antibodies to the gliadin fraction then I advise them to go off these foods for at least eight weeks and see if they feel better. What you need to observe are the advantages of avoiding certain foods and then notice how you react when you reintroduce them. If your symptoms clearly improve and you notice how bad you feel when you recommence your old habits you may find you are more motivated to adhere to your regimen. You should know that a lot of these intolerances hang around so you may have to change your habits for the long haul. It was only a few years ago that I discovered that I had a gluten intolerance by means of the above blood test. I had endured terrible skin problems including dermatitis and acne, tried every drug and cream known to man, visited countless medical practitioners and skin specialists, all to no avail. Having successfully treated a number of patients with skin conditions including acne, dermatitis and psoriasis by introducing gluten free diets and the appropriate vitamin and mineral supplements I decided it was time that I took a different look at my own problems. Much to my surprise my blood test was positive and once I initiated my own programme I noticed dramatic improvements in my skin condition and bowel function.

If all your tests are negative you might have to resort to the gold standard in order to discover whether you have any negative reactions to foods and this involves elimination and challenge. You can try this yourself if you wish and what you have to do is commence a very elementary diet including such foods as pear, white meat and rice and then introduce the substances that you may be reacting to one at a time and see how you respond. As this can be a rather elaborate procedure it is best that you consult with an expert in this area who can provide you with the appropriate guidance along the way.

2. Eliminate candida overgrowth. This syndrome is caused by an overgrowth of yeast germs in the bowel and typical symptoms include sugar cravings, excess flatulence, fungal and yeast infections as well as thrush, irritability, fatigue and nasal congestion aligned with a positive antibody test to candida albicans. Candida can be caused by excessive emotional stress, treatment with antibiotics or steroids, eating lots of sugary or yeast based foods and exposure to mouldy environments.

A yeast and sugar-free diet, acidophilus supplementation and herbal remedies including pau d'arco, cats claw, olive leaf extract, citrus seed, oregano and barberry taken for ten to twelve weeks can lead to the eradication of candida overgrowth but sometimes this treatment needs to go on for a much longer period of time. Anti-fungal medications such as nystatin, nizoral and diflucan may also need to be incorporated if these herbal remedies prove to be ineffective. Your response to treatment is monitored by the reduction of your symptoms and your candida antibody levels. Once these are substantially diminished, you are over the hurdle of managing candida, which in my experience is not always that easy.

3. Boost your digestive enzymes. As we get older our bodies produce less digestive juices and if you are suffering from burping and bloating chances are you are deficient. There are a number of tonics you can use to enhance your digestive enzymes ranging from simple water and lemon to the more potent remedies such as Swedish bitters, apple cider vinegar and aloe vera juice, which can also cleanse your bowel and stimulate elimination. If you have symptoms you should take these before meals at least twice a day and there's probably no harm in utilising these potions for extended periods of time.

4. Ensure you have adequate supplies of good germs in your bowel. Like digestive enzymes the germs that promote bowel health decline with age. American expert Natasha Trenev has been involved in a life-long study about the beneficial effects of certain strains of bacteria including what she calls super strains. These include Lactobacillus acidophilus NAS super strain, Bifidobacteria bifidum Malyoth super strain and Lactobacillus bulgaricus LB-51 super strain. In her book 'Probiotics Nature's Internal Healers' she explains why these super germs are so proficient at dealing with yeast infections and other disease-causing micro-organisms, protecting us against cancer, improving chronic constipation, helping us digest, boosting our immune systems and generally being the best ally any vulnerable digestive tract could wish for. I would strongly recommend that you incorporate these protective substances in your daily regimen. The ideal way is to take these with your morning meal.

5. Treat 'leaky gut' or increased intestinal permeability. Normally the lining of your bowel is intact and you only absorb what your body needs and eliminate the wastes. Like your ceiling the walls of your bowel can have tiny holes, which allow certain unwanted foreign particles to pass into your system. This means your bowel is leaking or has increased intestinal permeability. This not uncommon condition can lead to all sorts of health problems including arthritis, autoimmune diseases, migraines, mental fogginess and possibly even fatigue. It makes sense that your body would be weakened if you have to deal with an array of unwelcome visitors. Your doctor can perform a simple test on your urine, which assesses the presence of indican, a type of protein not normally present if you don't have 'leaky gut'. A positive test suggests that you have this condition and then it becomes important to investigate the underlying cause with food allergy, abnormal bowel germs, stress, alcohol, non-steroidal anti-inflammatory medication and chemotherapy being the most common instigators. Natural remedies such as aloe vera, slippery elm, glutamine and zinc can be used to repair the damaged gut lining. Clinical trials have also shown that selenium, vitamin A, docosahexaenoic acid found in fish oil, and lactoferrin, a type of protein with immune-enhancing properties, are effective treatments.

**Natural Remedies
Help to Repair Gut Lining**

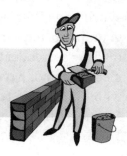

Putting theory into practice

I've indicated up to now that if fatigue is your primary concern you need to have those tests which assess your hormone levels, your vitamin status, food allergy or intolerance and you need to ensure that your digestive system, liver and adrenals are functioning to full capacity.

Stephen is a 40year-old architect who came to see me, having exhausted the medical roundabout. He had a long history of early morning fatigue, a layer of fat around his midriff, which had become extremely difficult to shed, eczema and irregular bowel habits which was most disconcerting. He was reluctant to tell me this but he only moved his bowels every 3-4 days. He'd had a series of blood tests, which were all normal. He tried a range of eczema creams and weight loss potions and as none of these made any difference he increasingly sort solace in the sweet anaesthetic that only alcohol can bring. When I saw him he was up to consuming at least 3-4 alcoholic drinks every night and was on a downward spiral.

Stephen's doctor was ready to prescribe antidepressants thinking that his morning lack of zip was an indicator that his brain chemistry was out of synch and all he needed was the right medication to get him up and running again. Stephen wasn't quite ready to surrender to the seductive promise of modern medicine and, having heard that I tend to look at the whole picture and do things a little differently came to see me. All I did was follow the basic principles that

I've already set out. Once I completed his hormonal panel I found without much surprise that his IGF-1, cortisol and DHEA levels were all low. His penchant for alcohol and the excess weight he was carrying would have undermined the performance of his liver where IGF-1 is produced. Having too much fat on the outside of your body also leads to the accumulation of fat around your liver. This results in what is called a 'fatty liver' which compromises the function of your liver cells which can reduce IGF-1 production. Stress would have taken its toll on his adrenals leading to diminished DHEA and cortisol levels.

Blood tests further showed that he had a gluten intolerance with raised anti-gliadin antibody levels suggesting that he should avoid foods containing wheat, rye, oats and barley, while his urine test was positive for leaky gut. He was also lacking in most of the B vitamins including vitamins B3, B6 and B12 as well as vitamin C, nutrients that support adrenal function. This was assessed by the functional questionnaire I mentioned earlier.

He also had a 'live blood cell' analysis and a biological terrain assessment test (BTA). These tests allow you to get up close and personal with the cells of your body. It's all very well having sufficient amounts of hormones and vitamins but what you really want to find out is how well your cells are functioning and how they are served by these vital substances. His 'live blood cell' test, which uses a small amount of blood that is viewed under a microscope to decipher the workings of your cells, confirmed that his liver was not up to scratch, his red cells had lost their capacity to deliver oxygen, his fat metabolism was inadequate, in fact he had excess fat in his blood stream and he was also carrying some abnormal critters around his body suggesting a yeast infection. His BTA, which utilises a urine, saliva and blood analysis to determine free radical levels, the acid/alkali balance of cells as well as liver, adrenal and kidney function, revealed that he had an excess accumulation of free radicals as well as an over-acidic cellular environment. Your cells function within an optimal acid/alkali range. Excessive acidity, which results from the over-consumption of acidic foods such as red meat, grains and alcohol can lead to your cells being too acidic which compromises their function.

In case you think that Stephen's picture is a disaster zone with cells that aren't working well, hormone and vitamin deficiencies, a digestive system, adrenal glands and liver that are struggling and food intolerance just for good measure, then I have to tell you that this state of affairs is not unusual. If you are suffering from fatigue, weight gain, skin problems, a poor memory and digestive complaints, you will discover that the underlying reasons for your difficulties are probably not that different from those of Stephen's. What's exciting about all of this is that these abnormalities and imbalances are all correctable.

We started off with rectifying his diet by eliminating gluten and yeast containing foods such as bread, mushrooms and alcohol. He was encouraged to increase his consumption of green vegetables and to limit his intake of red meat in order to reduce the acidity of his cells. We then proceeded to treat his yeast overgrowth with herbal compounds including pau d'arco, citrus seed extract and oregano that target excess yeasts and he also started taking a powder, containing aloe vera, glutamine, slippery elm and zinc, to treat his leaky gut.

To boost his adrenal function he commenced a formulation called Memozeal which includes herbs such as withania and gotu kola that modulate stress, and the vitamins B12 and folic acid for his memory. We attacked his low IGF-1 with trans-d tropin to increase growth hormone production.

Much to his delight and mine within 10 weeks his energy had improved. His cortisol and IGF-1 levels were up, his yeast overgrowth and leaky gut condition had diminished and his eczema was less troubling. His free radical score had gone down and his cells were less acidic. However he had only lost three kilos of weight. I encouraged him to return to some form of regular exercise, suggested that he reduce his carbohydrate intake, and introduced further energy boosters including coenzyme Q10 and a B vitamin complex. Four months later he was feeling much better. His energy levels continued to increase, his bloating had vanished, his eczema only flared-up if he had dietary transgressions, he had lost eight more kilos and his mental function was the best it has been in a long time. Overall he was very pleased with the progress he had made and was highly motivated to continue with his programme.

Joanne is a 52 year-old accounts executive

suffering from hot flushes, poor libido, dry skin and low back pain. Her brain wasn't functioning as well as she was used to as she struggled through her average working day and she was also concerned that her 'shrinking and sagging' breasts as she described them were a stark reminder that the sands of time were catching up with her. She used to be an exercise fanatic and even ran the occasional marathon but was beginning to find any form of exercise a daunting prospect.

Joanne's hormonal status was low with deficiencies in oestrogen, progesterone, cortisol, testosterone and DHEA as well as thyroid hormones and IGF-1. She was lacking in vitamin A, vitamin B3, vitamin C and the essential fatty acids. Her blood tests indicated that she had candida overgrowth and she also had a positive leaky gut test on urinalysis. While her 'live blood cell' test was quite reasonable, her BTA indicated that her free radicals were getting the better of her and her cells were too acidic which are common findings.

To pep up her hormones she started a replacement regimen including triest 1mg (this combines the three major female hormones oestradiol, oestrone and oestriol) DHEA 10mg, testosterone1mg and progesterone100mg taken in the form of a troche which is allowed to melt inside the cheek (see chapter 6). This is a nice and easy way to deliver all the hormones in one hit and it can also serve the purpose of stimulating growth hormone production. As her thyroid function was only minimally reduced she opted to supplement with kelp, which is a good source of iodine that the thyroid gland can use to make more hormones. To treat her candida overgrowth she commenced an acidophilus complex, which has the capacity to neutralise excess yeasts, as well as the herbs that Stephen took, and we replaced all the nutrients she was lacking. In order to fight those relentless free radicals she commenced the major league antioxidants; acetyl-L-carnitine, alpha-lipoic acid and coenzyme Q10 together with vitamin E and selenium.

After three months she returned with the happy news that her energy had taken a major upswing, her hot flushes were no longer troubling her and her long lost libido was staging a significant comeback. Although she was not quite there yet her enthusiasm for exercise had been rekindled and she was contemplating a return to a training regimen that had become a distant memory. All her hormones were operating at very respectable levels. Her free radical status had improved and her cells were less acidic. As far as her candida problem was concerned this took a while to manage and it was only after nine months that this problem receded into the background. One year later she has maintained her programme and is extremely keen to stay with her hormone and antioxidant regimen.

Stephen's and Joanne's experience is something I encounter daily in my practice. I see many unfortunate people who are washed-out and dried-up, who have lost their spark, who can't sleep and can't function and are offered medical solutions like anti-depressants and sleeping pills, which are utterly inappropriate because they fail to examine the underlying reason for these problems. Once your hormones and vitamins are measured together with the other necessary tests it's very easy to get a very clear idea where your deficiencies lie and from there it's not rocket science to institute the correct management which can restore the balance and energy that you are lacking.

Because insomnia and depression are intimately connected with fatigue and are often treated with medications that are associated with such awful side effects, it is well worth exploring how you can deal with these by utilising hormones and vitamins and other more natural methods.

BEATING THE INSOMNIA BLUES

Aside from eroding our energy levels if we don't sleep well, our immune systems suffer, we think and remember less clearly and we don't produce enough of those hormones such as melatonin and growth hormone that help us to stay young and healthy. Both melatonin, which is a hormone that regulates your sleep wake cycle and is a powerful antioxidant in its own right, and growth hormone are manufactured predominantly when you sleep. You probably didn't know this but if you deprive someone of sleep for more than a week they will die. We need sleep more than we need food. Just how much sleep we need is still up for debate and clearly some of us can survive on less. Most experts agree that around eight to nine hours will suffice.

The difficulties that we have don't simply reside in the nighttime hours. When our sleep does become disturbed it's what's happening during the day that has such an impact. If I had to identify the common denominator that unifies just about everyone's tribulations then a very simple dragon would be the primary enemy. Stress or rather the way we deal with it is the biggest hurdle. The more jangled our nerves are during the day the harder it is to relax when we want to go to sleep. In truth we all have stress. It's how we go about managing it that has such an effect on whether we rest easy at night. What stress does is to disturb the normal function of our adrenal glands. When our adrenals are in balance and we are dealing effectively with stress peaceful sleep becomes a much easier prospect.   If you find your mind is excessively active when you lie down at night so that it takes you a devilishly long time to fall asleep then stress may be the culprit. Waking up between three and four in the morning and then finding it an onerous task to settle down into any restful pattern means that unresolved tension is playing havoc with your nervous system. Managing stress isn't always that easy as you've no doubt discovered. Here are some directives for overcoming the dragon.

Dealing effectively with stress.

- Slow down, take your time. You have more time than you think. Eat more slowly, drive in the slow lane to work. Take time to savour this beautiful world in which we live: smell the flowers, stand in awe and gaze at the incredible sight of the ocean bathed in the powerful glow of the sun's rays, notice the trees and the cloud formations. Once you access the power, and I know that you will, the negative effects of stress will start to dissipate. You will have oceans of time to do whatever you want. Be patient. This transformation might not happen instantaneously.

- Introduce meditation into your daily regimen. Simply focussing on your breathing is one way to give your brain a rest from all that incessant activity. Learning a meditation technique such as transcendental meditation and practising this method for a mere twenty minutes daily will have anti-stress benefits. What meditation does is to increase your body's natural production of DHEA, which is known to improve feelings of well-being.
- Eat less carbohydrates. This will encourage your pancreas to produce less insulin which in turn gives cortisol, your stress hormone, a breather. Your body needs oxygen, water, protein in beans, fish, eggs and lean meat as well as essential fats found in nuts, seeds and oils and finally fruit and vegetables. Carbohydrates located in bread, cereals, potato, rice and pasta are not essential.
- Take herbal remedies. Herbs such as withania, gotu kola, Siberian ginseng, rehmania and oats will realign your adrenal glands and soothe your frazzled nervous system. The brain boosting formulation Memozeal has been formulated with this in mind. You need to give herbal tonics a while to work, as the benefits are often subtle and cumulative. These are taken during the day rather than at night. Expect positive results within four to six weeks
- Do some form of exercise in the early evening. This may involve going for a walk or a jog or even going to the gym and having a formal workout.

Exercise helps to release all that pent up tension and if you do this 4-5 hours before you go to sleep your mind should be ready to enjoy peaceful rest.

Nurture positive relationships

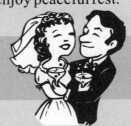

- Nurture positive relationships and resolve conflicts. Positive relationships generate those brain chemicals that help you sleep better. What I constantly notice is the amount of negativity going around whether it be in the news or what people say to each other. You can change this dynamic by being complimentary as often as possible without being dishonest or sickly sweet. Most of us love to hear nice things about ourselves and one way to receive positive strokes is to start dishing them out.
- Get a pet. If human affiliations aren't your forte then a loving relationship with a pet can be extremely comforting to the nervous system. I needn't tell you that a pet's love is unconditional. They love your smells - all of them.
- Have a break. This doesn't have to be in an exotic location. Any change from your normal routine will do and indulge yourself as often as possible.
- Enjoy a massage. Stress often leads to tight neck muscles that manifest as those searing headaches, which are classic sleep disruptors. A therapeutic

or deep tissue massage is what you need to relieve all those knots and reduce your tension. If you can, have such a massage at least once a month.

- Phosphatidylserine, which is derived from soya lecithin, has been shown to inhibit production of cortisol, the stress hormone. If your adrenals are producing too much cortisol this usually means that stress is the number one cause and reducing this hormone is one way to put a lid on the effects of excessive stress.

Now that you are on the road to mastering your stress you might need a little extra assistance to provide you with a substantial night's sleep. Here I would encourage you to resist using medication unless the natural remedies are not working for you. My favourites for inducing sleep are magnesium, melatonin, and the herbal remedies. I'm a great fan of magnesium and though there's not a lot of research on the effects of this mineral on sleep it does have a calming effect on the nervous system. As green vegetables and nuts, not the usual dietary staples, are the major sources of magnesium many of us would probably be lacking in this nutrient. If you suffer from any of the following symptoms you may have a magnesium deficiency. These include palpitations or an irregular heartbeat, cramps in your calf muscles, twitchy legs especially at night, constipation, lower backache when you get up in the morning or disturbed sleep. Taking magnesium earlier in the day and then in the evening is one way to address these problems and give your nervous system the respite it needs.

Melatonin, for those who are not familiar with this hormone, is produced predominantly in the pineal gland, which is located in your brain. If you place your finger just above the bridge of your nose you will be homing in on the site of this gland. In my first book 'Eternal Health' I gave melatonin huge plaudits as one of the primary anti-ageing hormones. There are some experts who argue that to talk about any hormone having anti-ageing properties is a touch premature at this stage but they could not dispute the mountain of research which shows that melatonin is a mighty powerful antioxidant. As a sleep restorer melatonin comes into its own. I'm not overly keen on using melatonin when your body is producing enough of this hormone and although research is being conducted on the very young my sense is that you should only look at regular nighttime supplementation after the age of 35. Having said that, I have one patient in his early thirties in a very high-powered job who found that regular sleep was eluding him. Having tried various potions he discovered melatonin, which proved to be the answer and he wasn't game to spend a night without it.

Progesterone is another sleep inducer. Men can also utilize this hormone if they are struggling to get a good night's rest. For women a reasonable dose would be 10-20mg of progesterone cream applied to the forearm ½ hour before bedtime while for men 5-10mg might help. As progesterone is the major female hormone that is produced in the second half of the menstrual cycle it might be unwise to utilise this hormone in the first part of the cycle.

As far as herbal tonics are concerned you have a wide variety to choose from and each herbalist will have their tried and trusted remedy. My preference is valerian, a herb that most of you might be familiar with, and hops - a lesser-known botanical, which also targets stress, tension and anxiety. The beauty of taking herbs is that they help you to sleep without any after-effects the next day.

Managing insomnia effectively

- Eat a high-carbohydrate meal at night. This will increase the production of an amino acid called tryptophan, which ultimately makes more melatonin.
- Make sure there is a two to three hour gap between your evening meal and when you go to sleep. Trying to sleep on a full stomach will make it more difficult for you to enjoy a relaxing night's sleep.
- Drink herbal teas such as chamomile towards the end of the day. This will encourage you to wind down and ease your mind into a more restful state.
- Do not indulge in caffeine, alcohol or cigarettes towards bedtime. These are stimulants.
- Use essential oils to enhance relaxation. Placing a few drops of clary sage, lavender and cedarwood on an aromatherapy vaporiser or in an oil burner an hour before you go to sleep will introduce a tranquil environment to your bedroom.
- Magnesium can be taken in a chelated form or as magnesium diglycinate. You should aim at 500mg daily in divided doses, morning and night time.
- Take valerian and hops one hour before you go to bed. A reasonable dose of valerian is an extract, which is equivalent to 2grams of the dry root while that of hops would be 350mg of the fruit of this herb.
- Before you start taking melatonin have your levels measured and the way to do this is via a salivary test sampled at night. You want to make sure that you do not expose your body to an excess amount

of any hormone as this may have detrimental effects in the long term. A good dose to start off with is 1mg taken two hours before sleep and if this doesn't work 3mg may be the quantity that you are looking at. I have a 1mg per decade rule. If you are in your forties 1-3 mg should be your limit. In your fifties you can increase this to 4mg and this goes up to 5mg once you hit sixty. When you take melatonin you will notice that you have the most vivid and exciting dreams. Some of my patients get a real kick out of this and when I take melatonin I find the technicolor nature of my dreams quite entertaining. If this is not a pleasurable experience for you, you may have to cut back on your dose, which should make your dreams more palatable.

- Progesterone cream 20mg for women and 5-10mg for men applied ½ hour before bedtime.

TARGETING DEPRESSION

I didn't know this but apparently depression is the second most common medical complaint in the USA and in that country only 25% of patients are treated adequately. There might be good reasons for this, as you will discover below. Overcoming this murky demon can prove to be very exhausting. While I'm not wishing to relegate psychotherapy, anti-depressants, healthy self-esteem, nurturing relationships, good genes and the complexity of this condition to the side lines, exploring hormonal and vitamin deficiencies might lead to dramatic improvements, especially when all the other options have been examined.

> ## This approach is intended for the management of mild to moderate depression.
>
> - Have your levels of B12 and folic acid measured. I find that many of my patients have sub-optimal levels of vitamin B12. This vitamin is important for the synthesis of serotonin, the brain chemical, which prevents depression. With ageing absorption of these nutrients diminishes.
> - Low levels of certain key hormones can lead to depression. These include testosterone, thyroid hormone, DHEA and oestrogen. Studies indicate that taking these hormones can alleviate depression especially if your levels are low.
> - Omega-3 fatty acids in the form of fish or flaxseed oil can also be utilised to manage depression. These improve the communication between nerve endings by making these more receptive to brain chemicals such as serotonin.
> - Clinical trials have yielded positive results with the herb st john's wort for managing mild to moderate depression. A recent study has even shown that this herb is superior to the medication paroxetine for managing severe depression without all the nasty side-effects.
> - S-adenosylmethionine also known as SAMe is a type of protein that is made in the body. There is some evidence that this nutrient can be used effectively to treat depression.
> - If your levels of magnesium and the B group vitamins are low, especially vitamin B3, then

supplementing with these might help.
- Tryptophan and 5-hydroxytryptophan are other natural remedies that can be used to overcome this debilitating condition. These operate by increasing serotonin in your brain.

You can see why conventional treatments might be missing the boat some of the time. If you are depressed for no reason then exploring the above might bring welcome relief. However you have to be cautious with this approach. These options should not be implemented without the guidance of your doctor. It is not a good idea to cease any form of anti-depressant medication and simply commence these suggestions. These remedies should not be added to your treatment as you might experience rather unpleasant symptoms.

Finally there is chronic fatigue syndrome (CFS). We still remain pretty much in the dark about this grossly misunderstood disorder. Medical wisdom still talks about cognitive behavioural therapy as if you could change the course of events by thinking or behaving this syndrome away. I don't pretend to have the final answer but here are some possibilities that might make a difference:

Managing CFS

- Almost certainly low hormone levels play their part. Growth hormone, DHEA, cortisol, testosterone, melatonin and thyroid hormone should be evaluated and treated if reserves have dwindled.

- Some experts view CFS as an energy production problem located in the mitochondrion, which is the battery that charges your cells. All the B vitamins, Vitamins C and E, magnesium, selenium, coenzyme Q10 and alpha-lipoic acid can be used to kick start your mitochondria. Encouraging evidence from scientific studies demonstrates that supplements of NADH (nicotinamide adenine dinucleotide), which helps to produce energy in the mitochondrion, and L-carnitine, have the capacity to reduce fatigue.

- Food intolerance/allergy, 'leaky gut' and an imbalance of bowel germs might be implicated. Treating candida overgrowth and eliminating gluten intolerance is important. Ask your doctor to order a comprehensive digestive stool analysis via a lab that does this type of test. This will give you a good overview of your bowel function.

- Poor sleep patterns need to be corrected. See the relevant section in this chapter. Other remedies that can be used to induce healthy sleeping habits include the nutrient L-theanine derived from green tea and the herb passionflower.

- One of the liver's major functions is to detoxify. This might be compromised. A caffeine clearance is one of the ways to assess liver detoxification capacity, as a routine blood test might not always identify imperfect liver function. Nutrients such as N-acetylcysteine, methionine and pine bark extract assist with liver function as do the herbs st mary's thistle, green tea extract, and globe artichoke.

- Infection is thought to play a part in the initiation of CFS. Antibiotics have been used in this regard. Natural alternatives include the herbs echinacea, astragalus and citrus seed extract, supplementary zinc and vitamin A and the nutrients lactoferrin and colostrum.

To balance the immune system which is thought to be out of line in CFS, omega-3 fatty acids, thymic protein A, which augments the function of the thymus where immune cells are manufactured, chlorella, reishi and shiitake mushrooms and phytosterols can be incorporated.

There is an excellent book on CFS edited by two Belgian experts doctors Englebienne and de Meirlier available via the website www.crcpress.com which investigates all the complexities underlying this crippling disease. Included in the factors that are thought to lead to this disease are heavy metals such as mercury, lead, cadmium and nickel, organophosphates, longstanding physical and mental stress, viral and bacterial infections, immune imbalance, allergies, pregnancy and exposure to radiation. Treatments that they propose include ampligen, an anti-viral and immune modulating agent that is administered by intravenous injection, which achieved some success in their trials, treatment with antibiotics, injections of vitamin B12 and folic acid and NADH. Growth hormone and DHEA also get a mention as possible treatments.

This book can be medically and technically demanding as it is not designed to be easily digestible by the layman but it does provide very useful information and lots of good insights. I thoroughly recommend it to anyone with an interest in this terrible disease.

Obviously managing CFS is a complicated business that regrettably does not always yield positive outcomes. If you are going to avail yourself of the above therapies you should locate a physician who is familiar with this approach.

Beating The Battle of The Bulge

Weight loss can be extremely difficult. We are programmed to store fat not lose it. Once you try to lose weight you will encounter all sorts of obstacles, as you are probably aware. It's not your fault if you can't lose weight or effectively maintain weight loss. Your evolutionary history, your cravings and easy access to foods that are rich in fats and sugars, your hormones that are out of balance making you hungry and insatiable are all factors that make weight loss a massive ordeal. I know I've been there. Although I've never been excessively overweight and I hope those of you who are in the unfortunate position of having substantial amounts of weight to lose won't feel insulted I'm going to let you into a secret. I have about six kilos of weight to lose. In the past year I've developed a little bit of extra flab around my middle, which is not that noticeable to others but I'm certainly aware of it. Up till now I've resorted to sucking my stomach in when I look at myself in the mirror and I haven't really put in a determined effort to shed myself of this spare tyre. Sure I have a healthy diet and exercise regularly but this has not resulted in any significant change in the abdominal area.

I decided that when I started to write this chapter would be a good time to put my money where my mouth is and so I'm now expending a considerable amount of effort to lose weight. And I'm sure it's not news to a lot of you that it's not easy. I now have to go about my day in a different way and change is not pleasant. Especially when it involves altering my eating habits. Here's another bit of self-disclosure of which I'm not proud. I love carbohydrates and sweet foods. Give me some chocolate mousse and I'm in alimentary heaven. Chocolate actually switches on that part of your brain which elicits feelings of pleasure and contentment. No doubt the chocolate manufacturers know about this. I'm sure I don't have to tell you that chocolate is also rich in fats and sugars which is a sure-fire way to increase that good old abdominal girth. So the other night when I attended a lavish banquet to celebrate my nephew's birthday and a rich chocolate mud cake presented itself in front of my gaping eyes I exercised self-restraint and did not allow a morsel of this delicious fare to pass my lips. How I overcame this seemingly irresistible temptation I will tell you shortly.

As I've already indicated our bodies don't like to lose weight. We are actually programmed to maintain or gain weight but once we decide that we want to embark on a weight loss programme our bodies will fight us every inch of the way. Way back when we were foraging for foods, and there were times of scarcity our cells learned to store fat in order to provide us with a ready source of energy so that we could survive. This genetic blueprint for survival has persisted to this very day so that when you start to lose weight you brain will tell you to eat more, your cells will resist fat loss and to top this all off your metabolism will slow down so that you will burn less fuel. What's even worse is that the quicker you lose weight the more your body will shut down so that when you hit the wall or come off your diet you may regain the weight that you have lost plus the bonus of a few added kilos. Does this sound like it's all a bit too hard? What we have to do is find a way to outsmart our recalcitrant genes. Here's the uplifting part. If like many others out there you're struggling to rid yourself of those unwanted kilos and more importantly to sustain weight loss then there just might be a way to make this process more manageable for you.

The comforting and sobering news is that you're not alone. Right now we're in the midst of a global obesity epidemic that has massive ramifications for healthcare delivery throughout the world. More often than not obesity leads to diabetes and with this potentially lethal disease comes a dramatic escalation in the incidence of heart attacks, strokes and even cancer. It's paradoxical that we are encouraged to consume and yet we are obsessed with being thin. We are a fat society yearning for the perfect body. And we're getting fatter by the minute. The increasing availability of foods that are perfect combinations of sugar and fat cleverly designed to fuel our desire to eat more, as well as our sedentary lifestyle, do not make things easier. More alarmingly our children are becoming flabbier and this can lead to a lifetime battle to beat the bulge. It you start off on the wrong footing the odds are really loaded against you. As you get older you also tend to put on weight. Incredibly in the USA the average adult stacks on one pound per year between the age of twenty-five and fifty which constitutes a substantial weight gain. Around menopause there is also a tendency to lose muscle and gain fat that can lead to an apple shape appearance, which is more

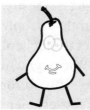 Better to look like a pear then an apple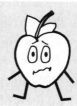

typical of the masculine body type when things go belly up. It is this fat that sits in the middle of your frame that is synonymous with the now famous syndrome X or the metabolic syndrome as it is sometimes known. The more characteristic female pear shape may be unsightly in the eyes of some resulting in a never-ending obsession with shedding that dreaded cellulite but it is not the fat residing in this area that generates a health risk. Syndrome X defines a cluster of metabolic aberrations including high triglycerides, a form of fat that can trigger heart disease, low HDL, which is the cholesterol that is thought to unblock your blood vessels, and high blood pressure. All of this is thought to result from excess weight around the waistline with the hormone insulin occupying a central role in this metabolic saga.

Insulin is responsible for opening up the door so that glucose can get into your cells. When you eat pasta or rice or cereal these foods are broken down into the glucose that enters your blood stream ready to be utilised by your cells for the purpose of providing you with the energy you need. Your pancreas sees to it that you have enough insulin to make glucose available to you. Once you have a lot of fat around your middle this process ceases to operate in an efficient fashion. It is this fat that gets in the way of insulin function so that a condition known as insulin resistance results. This means that your glucose will find it more and more difficult to move into your cells. When this happens, instead of burning fat you will conserve this energy resource and your body will go into fat storage mode. To put it simply obesity leads to insulin resistance and insulin resistance begets obesity. There's this terribly judgemental misconception that people who are overweight are slothful and simply aren't trying hard enough to lose weight. This is not true. When you're overweight your physiology makes it even more difficult for you to lose weight. Because your body becomes less efficient at generating energy from the fuel supplies that you have you'll be compelled to eat more. Is it any wonder that your waistline is expanding? In short your metabolism has gone into reverse gear and one of the ways you can beat this is to adopt a scientific approach. Your doctor can perform a blood test, which measures your insulin and glucose levels before and after you've had a sugar drink in order to determine whether you have insulin resistance. A fasting insulin level of 10 or more strongly suggests that you have this problem. What we need to do is find a way to interrupt this vicious cycle. This is where hormones and vitamins might be able to turn this whole catastrophe around. Let's start off with the hormones in sequence to see how this might be possible.

GROWTH HORMONE

There is no question that growth hormone has the ability to increase muscle mass and to burn fat. Studies also indicate that growth hormone performs even better when accompanied by an exercise programme and dietary changes. (1) This tells us that you cannot rely on growth hormone alone to facilitate weight loss. You need to be exercising and eating differently as well. There is one problem with incorporating growth hormone. In the short term this hormone can make insulin resistance worse but if you follow your exercise and eating plan you can prevent this from happening. Once you start to build muscle as a consequence of growth hormone treatment then your cells will start to respond appropriately to insulin and you will find it easier to lose weight. Fat gets in the way of growth hormone production and the fatter you are the less growth hormone your body will produce. However when you start to lose all this fat you will restore your body's natural ability to manufacture growth hormone, which will reduce your need for any growth hormone supplementation.

If your body is producing enough growth hormone it's probably unwise to entertain the thought of using this hormone. However if your levels are low then you should consider incorporating growth hormone to help you with your weight loss programme. You need to do this in conjunction with your doctor who will measure your IGF-1 levels in order to establish whether you have sufficient growth hormone present.

TESTOSTERONE

Almost universally studies show that testosterone helps men to build muscle and lose fat. This is especially the case if testosterone levels are low. Insulin works more efficiently and glucose becomes much more available once testosterone is operating at maximal capacity. Like it does for growth hormone, excess fat reduces testosterone. Similar principles therefore apply. Taking testosterone is a temporary measure helping your body to build muscle and lose fat, restoring your insulin function, which also makes it easier for you to burn fat, and renewing your body's ability to provide you with healthy supplies of testosterone. However you should only consider testosterone treatment if your levels are low. It would be unwise to take testosterone if your body is churning out reasonable amounts of this hormone.

With regard to the female experience, testosterone can pose problems. Although this hormone is a muscle builder having too much testosterone can lead to insulin resistance in the female body and it is thought that this kind of imbalance, which can happen around menopause, might lead to the typical masculine type of weight gain experienced by some women. In other words if you are developing that bulge around the middle have your hormones checked. Your body might be dealing with an excess of testosterone. This is true of polycystic ovarian syndrome, which is characterised by weight gain and the development of those features associated with high levels of testosterone such as unsightly facial hair and acne. Interestingly here insulin resistance appears to be the driving force behind this metabolic disorder indicating that both an abundance of testosterone and an overflow of insulin can have adverse consequences for women.

OESTROGEN AND PROGESTERONE

Oestrogen and progesterone can improve insulin sensitivity and help with weight loss. However, having too much of these hormones can in fact compromise insulin function and lead to weight gain. (2)(3) I have found (in my practice) that while some of my patients are very satisfied with their hormone treatment others experience bloating and weight gain. By reducing the dosage these problems seem to sort themselves out. Having worked in this area for a while now I have come to realise that low dose replacement with oestrogen and progesterone, which elevate hormone levels to the middle of the range, leads to the most effective weight loss.

DHEA AND CORTISOL

DHEA works wonders with laboratory animals. They lose weight and they run around like fit, healthy and happy gym junkies as if they were at a health resort. In humans DHEA improves insulin sensitivity and taking this hormone might assist with weight loss if your levels are low and you are suffering from insulin resistance. DHEA also has the capacity to make testosterone in women and oestrogen in men and this is not always a desirable outcome. Remember excessive amounts of testosterone can promote insulin resistance in women and too much oestrogen is not good for the male prostate. To derive the maximum benefit from DHEA this can be prevented and I will outline how this can be achieved in the menopause chapter.

Although we need cortisol to provide us with our basic energy and drive having too much of this hormone shuts the door on insulin. Have you ever heard of Cushing's disease? These poor folk have chronically elevated levels of cortisol leading to obesity and diabetes all because of the negative impact that cortisol has on insulin. Stress generates cortisol. If you suffer from ongoing stress then your body will keep providing you with cortisol. Have you ever noticed that when you are stressed for an extended period of time and you don't eat you don't lose weight? This is because all that cortisol tells your insulin to take a holiday as your body gets the message that you are heading into a famine. The result is that you preserve your fat stores. In other words unrelenting stress is your body's enemy. No wonder we all find it so easy to gain weight and so difficult to achieve the opposite.

How do you master cortisol? DHEA can help you. That's why meditation is good for you. It increases DHEA, neutralises cortisol and has the potential to help you lose weight. The nutrient phosphatidylserine which is derived from soy can also decrease cortisol levels.

THYROID HORMONE

Your metabolism depends on thyroid hormone. If your body is not producing sufficient thyroid hormones your metabolism will slow down and it will become easier for you to gain some weight. The real drama starts to unfold when you lose weight. This is when your thyroid starts to shut down as your body thinks once again that you are heading into times of scarcity and it's time to batten down the hatches in order to deal with what appears to be a long period of starvation. As we said before you are programmed to preserve your weight. Weight loss flies in the face of your body's natural inclination. If you've lost some weight and you've hit the wall and no matter what you do you can't seem to get your body to go any further or you simply can't initiate any weight loss at all this would be a good time to have your thyroid hormone levels measured especially if you've noticed that you have cold hands and feet and you feel sluggish and slow which are classical indicators of thyroid hormone deficiency. Low thyroid hormones lead to cravings for carbohydrates which incidentally also occur if you are deficient in B vitamins and magnesium. I usually commence thyroid hormone treatment when levels are sub-optimal. My preference is Armour thyroid treatment with the starting off dose being 30mg daily in the morning before breakfast. The equivalent amount of compounded physiologic sustained release thyroid extract is an alternative option. Depending on the response to treatment the dose can be increased to as much as 90mg daily. This form of therapy does not have to go on indefinitely as I often find I can taper or discontinue Armour thyroid once weight loss is successfully achieved.

MELATONIN

Melatonin is better known for its ability to treat jet lag and insomnia but now it also appears that this hormone can be included in a weight loss programme. Rats are less exposed to the weight provoking effects of excess cortisol and even find it easier to lose weight when treated with melatonin. Wouldn't it be nice if we took this hormone to alleviate insomnia and we discovered that we weighed less in the morning?

VITAMINS AND SPECIAL NUTRIENTS

There is a huge amount of hype and hard sell that surrounds products purported to guarantee quick weight loss. Unfortunately the sales pitch usually exceeds any natural product's capacity to deliver. The scientific research that substantiates the claims that are made is lacking in most instances. Aside from limited evidence, which shows that drinking a lot of green tea will help you to burn fat and taking large amounts of 5-hydroxytryptophan, which is a type of protein, will promote a sensation of satiety there isn't a lot to get excited about.

There are however a group of vitamins and other nutrients that can help to improve insulin function and together these substances might make it easier for you to lose weight. What these products do is to make your cells more responsive or sensitive to insulin allowing glucose a smoother transit into your cells. This in turn might make fat burning a more achievable proposition. These include the antioxidants alpha-lipoic acid and coenzyme Q10, the minerals chromium, zinc and magnesium, the herb cinnamon, the mineral vanadium, which is taken in the form of vanadyl sulphate and omega-3 fatty acids found in fish and flaxseed oil. Zinc and magnesium will only be effective if your levels of these minerals are low. This might also be true for chromium although I have found that my patients respond extremely well to this nutrient. Alpha-lipoic acid, coenzyme Q10 and vanadium can be taken twice daily in the morning and at lunchtime while the best time to take cinnamon is with your evening meal as this substance has the added benefit of lowering your cholesterol which is manufactured mostly while you sleep. This substance should be taken in the form of a powder.

Have you ever noticed that when you put on weight you become even more ravenous and you just can't stop eating? This is because you might be suffering from a phenomenon known as leptin resistance. Leptin is a hormone produced by our fat cells which tells us that we have eaten enough. Obese folk suffer from leptin resistance which means that their bodies don't tell them when to stop eating. This leads to increased hunger and compulsive eating. Omega-3 fatty acids might be the solution to this seemingly uncontrollable problem. Not only do these nutrients improve insulin sensitivity but they also seem to have the potential to reduce leptin resistance which would make you eat less. Aside from supplementing with omega-3 fatty acids the beneficial fats are also found in nuts, seeds, extra virgin olive oil and avocado.

To achieve the best effects chromium needs to be taken with each meal. The nutrients that I have found to be most effective are chromium and alpha-lipoic acid. I suggest you commence with these and add the others on the list in the order in which they appear below.

Improving insulin sensitivity

- Chromium chelate 200mcg three times daily
- Alpha-lipoic acid 200mg twice daily
- Cinnamon 1 gram at night
- Omega-3 fatty acids found in fish and flaxseed oil 1 gram daily
- Coenzyme Q10 100mg daily
- Vanadyl sulphate 75mg twice daily
- Zinc sulphate 15mg twice daily
- Magnesium diglycinate 300mg twice daily

Your response to these nutrients can be assessed by your insulin and glucose levels, which should come down over time. It should require less insulin to get the glucose into your cells. Your weight loss should coincide with this improvement.

EATING PLAN

Call it a diet, call it a lifestyle change or an eating plan. Whichever way you look at it you are going to have to change your eating habits for the long haul. This doesn't mean that you have to starve yourself. Losing weight in a hurry is not the answer as your body will soon get wise to this plan and will shut down rather rapidly which means that you will hit the wall and find it more difficult to continue with your programme. You will become despondent and you may start to resort to your old habits. Before you know it you have regained the weight you have lost and then some.

You have to be patient although this can be trying in a culture which embraces instant gratification and quick results. Ideally you should aim to lose not more than one kilogram every two weeks. This won't set off alarm bells in that part of your brain, which regulates your desire to eat as well as your metabolic rate. This can be achieved by reducing your carbohydrate and fat intake and eating more protein. High protein diets stimulate satiety which will prevent you from overconsuming. Your diet should be comprised mostly of vegetables, salads, some fruit, nuts, seeds, a fair amount of protein in the form of fish, eggs, white and lean meat and soy and a limited intake of grains provided you have no allergies to these foods.

This is in line with the low glycaemic index diet, which has the ability to stabilise your blood sugar leading to a more even insulin response. A low glycaemic index means these foods are converted into glucose more slowly in your body, which allows your insulin to function more efficiently and this in turn makes you crave less sugar and you end up eating less. When insulin is in the groove burning fat becomes an easier proposition. The green vegetables, legumes, apples, pears, cherries, peaches and basmati rice are examples of foods with a low glycaemic index. Potatoes, pumpkin, watermelon, sweet biscuits, corn chips and mars bars have a high glycaemic index. There is a very good book written by Australian expert on the glycaemic index Professor Jennie Brand Miller called 'The GI factor' which lists a range of foods with their glycaemic index and it would be worthwhile acquiring this book to become aware of all the foods you eat and where they rate with regard to their glycaemic index.

Here are the principal elements of this diet:

1. **Eat less than fifty grams of fat daily.**
   - A handful of nuts and seeds comprising cashews, almonds and sesame seeds = 25 grams of fat
   - One avocado = 20 grams of fat
   - One tablespoon tahini = 5 grams of fat
   - 1 tsp olive oil = 5 grams of fat
   - One fillet grilled fish = 2 grams of fat
   - One skinless chicken drumstick = 8 grams of fat

2. **Eat 100-130 grams of carbohydrate (cho) daily**
   - 2 cups of cauliflower = 15 grams of cho
   - 2 cups of broccoli = 15 grams of cho
   - 3 cups of spinach = 15 grams of cho
   - 2 tomatoes = 9 grams of cho
   - 1 head of iceberg lettuce = 10 grams of cho
   - 1/5 cup of cooked brown or white rice = 10 grams of cho

- 1 cup of cornflakes = 35 grams of cho
- 1 cup of puffed rice = 25 grams of cho
- 1 peach = 15 grams of cho
- 1 apple = 15 grams of cho
- 1 cup of blueberries = 14grams of cho

3. **Eat at least one gram of protein per kilogram daily**

- One skinless chicken breast = 10 grams of protein
- One average small lean portion of steak = 15 grams of protein
- One average fish fillet = 10 grams of protein
- One hundred grams of tofu = 18 grams of protein
- One egg = 8 grams of protein

Protein powders made from soy, rice or whey consumed with soy, low-fat dairy or rice milk can be a rich source of this nutrient. Having one of these drinks between meals is an ideal way to stop sugar cravings. Some protein powders, especially those containing fibre that stimulate the sensation of fullness, can be utilised as meal replacements in the early stages of your programme to help facilitate weight loss. This can be extremely helpful if you are finding it difficult to shed those stubborn fat cells.

4. Find out whether you have a candida or gluten allergy. Most of my patients who have a candida or yeast problem lose a substantial amount of weight when they embark on a yeast-free diet. I have a sense that we have become far too attached to grains in the form of bread, pasta, cereals and biscuits and

this has set us up to develop all sorts of allergies. What you crave is often what you are allergic to and it's especially the sweet foods that can lead to swings in your blood sugar, which would exacerbate insulin resistance. A yeast-free diet would allow you to interrupt this cycle and liberate you from your compulsive desire to eat foods that are high in sugar.

5.   Reduce your consumption of alcohol. Alcohol stimulates a hormone called ghrelin which promotes hunger and this will encourage you to eat more.   Incidentally your body also produces more ghrelin when you are trying to lose weight and ghrelin promotes leptin resistance.   Is it any wonder that this process is so awesomely difficult?

Don't be seduced by chocolate

6.   If you find that you are seduced by foods that overflow with fat and sugar such as the highly tempting chocolate mud cake that I mentioned at the beginning of this chapter do what I do and visualise all the disastrous consequences of giving in to such transient and wanton desire.   Imagining all the future pain that this indulgence will cause you might make this temporary pleasure less attractive.

HERE IS AN EATING PLAN WHICH CAN FORM THE NUCLEUS OF YOUR NEW DIET

Sample daily menu

BREAKFAST:

- Start the day with a glass of luke warm water with squeezed whole lemon to get your digestive juices flowing and make your system more alkaline.
- Poached eggs with one slice whole grain toast plus teaspoon olive oil or butter

or

- 1½ cups of corn flakes or muesli with low fat soy milk or rice milk combined with a handful of blueberries plus four strawberries. You can garnish this with ½ a handful of almonds, cashews and sesame seeds.

or

- Protein powder with either water or soy, rice or low fat milk.
- Midmorning snack: one apple or peach or a handful of cherries

LUNCH:

- One grilled fish fillet/ chicken breast or 100grams of tofu with a green salad or Greek salad plus ½ avocado
- Mid-afternoon snack: Protein drink with soy or rice milk or low fat cow's milk

EVENING MEAL:

- Stir fry tofu or chicken with mixed vegetables including broccoli, carrots, onions, cauliflower, spinach, celery and zucchini in olive oil

DESSERT:

- Mixed fruit including blueberries, cherries, apricots and pear with yoghurt.

Maintaining adequate hydration is also important. Undoubtably the healthiest liquid that should be passing your lips is water. Ideally you should drink five to six glasses of water daily, which is always a challenge for most of us. Tap water is a definite no-no, as you will be exposing yourself to an assortment of viruses, bacteria, pesticides, industrial chemicals and heavy metals such as lead and aluminium. Various forms of filtered water are available with the best system being the steam-distilled or reverse osmosis variety.

EXERCISE

Exercise is vital for weight loss. If you are not used to exercising you need to start somewhere. Walking is probably the easiest way to get into some form of routine. If you can find a place close to your home where the air is unpolluted and the environment is pleasant so much the better. What you need to build up to is a 45-60 minute walk at least five times a week, which generates a healthy sweat. If you are adept at counting your pulse sustaining a rate of 90-110 beats per minute for 45 minutes will place you in the fat burning zone. It may take you some time to reach this level so be patient with yourself and progress at your own pace.

Another way you can increase the amount of walking that you do is to resist using the elevator, or parking your car some distance from the shopping mall so that you are guaranteed of some extra exercise. Finding a friend to exercise with can make this activity more enjoyable and a fun experience but remember to keep your mind on the job at hand and don't dawdle. Aside from assisting with weight loss exercise improves insulin sensitivity, which further rewards your efforts. Regular exercise lowers your blood pressure, which is an added bonus for those who have problems in this area.

Finding a way to make your exercise a fun and joyous

activity will also help to make this a regular part of your daily routine. For example if you live near the beach walking along the sand and the water can be extremely invigorating and lots of fun. If you were to exercise in the outdoors enjoying the beauty and the nurturing qualities of nature wherever you go can make this activity truly pleasurable.

Another form of exercise that you need to consider is weight training. Having a firm and healthy muscle mass helps our old friend insulin and the more muscle you have the more fat you burn. Strong muscles build strong bones and when you consider that osteoporosis is a disease that threatens the ageing male almost as much as it does the female of the species staying in good condition assumes even greater proportions. Need I tell you that we live in a culture which is obsessed with a healthy physique? If ever there was an incentive to get into shape surely this must be it. It's never too late to commence such a programme and the best way to go about it would be to join a gym or employ a personal trainer to guide you in this new endeavour. You need to increase your weights periodically so that you are constantly promoting optimal muscle tone.

I've discovered an excellent tip from reading American health expert Oz Garcia's book entitled 'The Healthy High Tech Body' in which he suggests that instead of counting to seven when you lift a weight a better way would be to count to 14 on the way up and ten on the way down. This way you will be doing fewer repetitions but your muscle strength will improve demonstrably. You can also use this strategy to introduce heavier weights which will further contribute to building muscle mass. I've certainly found this to be the case and would encourage you to follow this approach. Weight training also encourages your body to produce more testosterone and growth hormone and we could always do with some more of those.

For those who are balking at the thought of beginning an exercise regimen which might seem like a laborious chore here's an inducement that might help you to jump into your lycra suit. Exercise will improve your sex life. You don't have to become an Olympic champion overnight. Start slowly and take your time to increase the amount of exercise that you do.

I would encourage you to enjoy a variety of exercise routines including stretching via yoga, weight training and jogging or power-walking. It all becomes easier once you establish a regular pattern of behaviour. Once exercise is a habitual part of your life you will be releasing those chemicals that reinforce persistent activity.

PUTTING IT ALL TOGETHER

So there you have it hormones, nutrients, diet and exercise. None of these is a magic elixir on its own but together they might just make it easier for you to lose weight. You would need to enlist the help of a physician who can measure your hormones and perform a blood test to see whether you are suffering from insulin resistance. If your hormones are low, commencing the appropriate treatment to boost these might just be the tonic you need to get you on the right track. Most women are of the impression that taking hormones will make them put on weight but this is not supported by scientific evidence. Lets have a look at how these principles can be applied in the real world.

How sally lost weight

Sally was a 53 year-old woman who had just gone through menopause. For the past 10 years she had steadily put on weight. She had tried various weight loss programmes and different forms of HRT but none of these helped her to lose weight or reduce her menopausal symptoms, which included hot flushes, dry skin, anxiety and depression. She was also suffering from high blood pressure for which she was taking medication.

When I saw her she was 20 kilos overweight. All her hormones were low except for testosterone, which was elevated because she was suffering from insulin resistance. Her liver enzymes were raised which often reflects the accumulation of fat around the liver. She commenced hormone treatment in the form of a troche (a lozenge which can be placed inside the cheek or under the tongue) combination, which included: triest ½ mg, (80% oestriol, 10% oestrone, 10% oestradiol) progesterone 50mg and DHEA 10mg. (a complete description of this type of treatment is found in chapter six) She took ½ of this troche twice daily. She also started Armour thyroid 30mg daily for one month, which she increased to two capsules daily for the second and third month. She also introduced dietary changes including a reduction of carbohydrates and commenced alpha-lipoic acid and chromium to improve her insulin sensitivity. She hadn't exercised for some months so we decided that this was a good time to reintroduce a walking programme.

When she returned three months later she was pleased to announce that she felt much better. She had lost 5 kilos, her moods had stabilised and she was able to reduce her blood pressure medication. Her hormone levels had gone up although there was still room for improvement. Her insulin levels had dropped dramatically and her liver enzymes had normalised. All in all a very satisfying result so far.

She stayed on her hormone and supplement regime and returned three months later. She was still feeling good and had lost another 3 kilos. Her hormone levels had continued to climb into a more acceptable range. Although her insulin resistance had lessened she was still suffering from this problem and her blood pressure was still high. We decided to keep going with her regimen as I felt that she was doing very well despite the fact that she still had a way to go. Much to my surprise she contacted me six weeks later and announced that she had stopped her hormone treatment as she thought that it was making her blood pressure go up and she was getting strange symptoms which included numbness in her legs and around her ears which she attributed to the hormone treatment. Despite my reassurance that it was unlikely to be the hormones that were causing any problems we agreed that she should stay off her treatment for another four weeks at which stage we would see how she was going.

When she walked into my practice I could see that she was markedly agitated and we discovered that her blood pressure had taken a considerable upswing. As she was discouraged she had stopped exercising. We recommenced her troches but this time at a slightly lower dose and she also increased her blood pressure medication and agreed to return to regular exercise. I saw her two months later and at that stage she was going well. She had sustained a weight loss of 10 kilos and had renewed enthusiasm for her programme. The moral of this tale is that if you're receiving hormone treatment, you're going well and then you start to develop uncomfortable and distressing symptoms all you might need is to have your treatment adjusted. I have seen this in my patients periodically. Once hormones are measured and the necessary changes are made then the programme can usually proceed quite smoothly with ongoing weight loss.

Anne, another one of my patients, had a strikingly similar story. She was a lady in her mid-forties and although she hadn't quite reached menopause yet her DHEA levels and thyroid function were low and she had started to put on some weight around her tummy. She was tired, depressed and had repeated bouts of bloating after meals. Her blood test indicated that she had a candida problem, which was the cause of her bloating and might also have contributed to her fatigue. She commenced DHEA, Armour thyroid, a yeast-free diet and herbal remedies targeting her candida overgrowth. It took a little while to adjust her DHEA and thyroid treatment to arrive at the right dose but once this was achieved she turned the corner, started to lose weight and felt much better. She has remained on a maintenance dose of DHEA and Armour thyroid and takes an assortment of vitamins and nutrients to sustain her throughout the day.

With regard to using troches as opposed to hormone creams swallowing a large proportion of hormones can compromise growth hormone levels which might in turn reduce muscle mass.   For those women who are finding it difficult to maintain their muscle tone and find that they are becoming flabby, using creams rather than troches might be a better option.

Henry was in his late 40's when he came to see me. He'd really let himself go and his frame had ballooned to a sizeable 125 kilos. His blood profile revealed that he had marked insulin resistance with high blood glucose levels and elevated cholesterol. Although he wasn't quite there yet he was staring down the barrel of diabetes and his testosterone levels were markedly diminished.   Henry had not exercised for some years so I suggested that he start a 15minute walk three times a week with his wife. The plan was to gradually increase the duration of this activity over the next three months.   He commenced a low carbohydrate diet and supplements for insulin resistance including cinnamon as his cholesterol was elevated, as well as chromium and alpha-lipoic acid. He also started testosterone replacement in the form of a 50mg troche taken in divided doses daily.

To prevent the formation of extra oestrogen, which can often happen with those who are overweight as the more fat cells you have the more oestrogen your body can produce, we included a medication called arimidex, which inhibits aromatase, at a dose of ½ mg twice weekly. Aromatase is the enzyme that converts testosterone to oestrogen and it's sometimes necessary to use arimidex when there is the threat of making excess oestrogen.

Henry stuck religiously with his programme and in the first six months lost a healthy 10 kilos. He continued his testosterone replacement and the rest of his regimen for another year after which he had lost a further 20 kilos. He had

15 more kilos to go to reach his goal weight and as his testosterone levels were beginning to escalate we decided it was time that he could go it alone without any hormone treatment. Once significant weight loss starts to occur healthy testosterone levels can be naturally restored. I was very satisfied with Henry's progress so I arranged an appointment for three months later to monitor his status. Disappointingly he returned having regained eight kilograms of weight. He was so close to his dream that he allowed his resolve to weaken and he had slid back into some of his bad eating habits. Equally he had allowed his daily exercise routine to slide. As his hormone levels were satisfactory I decided that what he needed was some encouragement rather than any major treatment change and I am pleased to announce that he is continuing to lose weight and at this point is pretty close to his original objective. When we last measured his glucose and insulin levels they had practically normalised. In terms of his metabolic profile and health status he is a million miles away from where he was when we began his programme two years ago. This is quite an achievement for someone who was that close to developing a serious disease like diabetes.

And how is my weight loss progressing? During the two weeks that it took me to write this chapter I lost one kilogram of weight, which puts me right on track and then the other night my mother's birthday came around and we went to this wonderful restaurant overlooking the Sydney harbour bridge. It took all the self-control that I could muster not to undo all that hard work in one evening.

Finally and without wishing to set you up for too much disappointment once you have unleashed your power and have discovered your passion and your purpose you will need to eat much less. Then your weight might drop off effortlessly. Wouldn't that be miraculous? Until that day happens utilising the strategies and the programme outlined in this chapter will help you to deal with what seems to be an insurmountable challenge.

There's this story about Abie and Sarah. Having lead a happy and eventful life with many a satisfying moment in their relationship Abie finally succumbs to the inequities of old age and shuffles off this mortal coil. After a six-month mourning period Sarah realises that she is missing Abie terribly and decides that this is a good time to re-establish some form of connection with the old rogue to see how he is getting on. So she goes to a séance and after some initial difficulties manages to hook up with her late husband. "So Abie," she enquires. "How are you getting on? What do you do with yourself the whole day?" 'Well," says Abie. "I get up in the morning and I have sex. Then I have something to eat and I have sex again. Then I rest for a short time and I have sex again. Then I have lunch and have sex and just before the evening meal I have sex again." "Wow", says Sarah, "so it's pretty good for you in heaven then." "Whose in heaven?" replies Abie. "I'm a rabbit in Denver, Colorado."

It's really sad to think that we have to wait before we reincarnate as a four-legged creature before we can enjoy unrestrained sexual expression. If you examine current sexual surveys you will find that a staggering 50% of adult females have simply lost interest in sex while a similar number of the opposite sex over the age of forty have some sort of problem rising to the occasion. (1) Although the act of sexual intercourse appears to be a rather simple exercise the intricate wiring set up in our brains and the complex array of chemicals and hormones that allow us to enjoy this endeavour has yet to be fully understood. What we do know is that sex is good for us. Sexually active people have fewer heart attacks, are less depressed and anxious, get sick less often and may even have a lower incidence of cancer. Endorphins released during orgasm can dull pain, which is useful for those who suffer from migraines or arthritis. Frequent orgasm has even been linked to a longer life. Without wishing to undo all the exercise related information that I presented to you in the previous chapter intercourse has the capacity to burn up to 200 calories in the space of a few minutes, which is the equivalent of a 15minute stint on the treadmill.

Undoubtably whether you are having a fulfilling sex life depends on the quality of the relationship with your partner but if desire, pleasure and enjoyment have evaporated and you can't understand why it would certainly be worthwhile exploring all those physical events that are responsible for making your sexual experience a happy one. Here is that state of our knowledge to date

THE HORMONES

GROWTH HORMONE

If I had a dollar for every male who consulted me complaining of the difficulties that he had with maintaining an erection then I would be a very rich man. It appears that there are a lot of men out there who don't have problems getting an erection but do find it hard to sustain their erection for an extended period of time. Aside from the new generation of Viagra-like medications, which facilitate erection on demand for up to 36 hours, growth hormone might appear to be the saviour that most men are seeking. A series of audacious experiments by a German research team who aspirated blood from the penile veins of a group of men suffering from erectile dysfunction (ED) and then compared these samples with those taken from a healthy group has revealed that growth hormone levels were significantly lower in the ED sufferers. (2) What growth hormone does is to increase a chemical called cGMP, which in turn allows the smooth muscle of the penis to relax thereby allowing for the influx of blood that establishes an erection. Viagra and its relatives also function by increasing cGMP. When the healthy subjects were aroused their growth hormone levels increased but this was not the case for the ED group. When this group did get erections the rise in growth hormone was much lower than that experienced by the healthy group.

Not only may growth hormone be responsible, at least in part, for the initiation of erections, claim these scientists, but it is the decline in growth hormone production with age that may contribute to some of the sexual problems that men have to deal with as they get older, including maintaining an erection. For any man who has low growth hormone levels and is struggling in this area boosting this hormone might be worth a shot.

TESTOSTERONE

For promoting desire testosterone is far and away the champion of all the hormones. For both sexes this hormone ignites libido or the eagerness to take matters to the next phase. Testosterone switches on a chemical in the brain called dopamine, which leads to those sexual urges that propel us into action. If you don't have any sexual feelings and you can't understand why, low testosterone levels might be responsible. Re-establish the flow of testosterone and the sexual fires might start to burn again. It has to be said that for women this relationship is more complex as not all studies have confirmed that testosterone is the answer for those women who experience low sexual desire. In fact for those women who want to restore their sexual passion it's far better to take testosterone in combination with oestrogen or at least ensure that the body is primed by sufficient amounts of oestrogen before replacing dwindling supplies of testosterone. When these two hormones are operating in tandem desire, sexual sensation and frequency of intercourse increase significantly.

While the presence of both of these hormones contributes to a healthy female genital tract it is testosterone that heightens the receptiveness of the female genitalia. Testosterone has been known to facilitate orgasm possibly by enhancing clitoral sensitivity. It's only necessary to advance testosterone to the middle of the normal range in order to experience the benefits. A reasonable dose of testosterone would be 0.5-1mg daily taken in the form of a troche or a cream in combination with the other hormones. Once this treatment is commenced regular monitoring of hormone levels is needed to ensure that healthy rations of this hormone are maintained.

If testosterone defines the essence of lust or libido can this hormone also be held responsible for driving erectile function? We've already learned that growth hormone contributes to the initiation and preservation of this vital activity so how necessary is testosterone? There is general agreement that a certain amount of testosterone is needed to facilitate penile erections but the experts are divided as to the critical nature of this hormone. There are as many studies supporting testosterone's primary responsibility for erectile function, as there are those that fail to establish an association between this hormone and erectile dysfunction. (3)(4) To cut a long story short, if you are having trouble either getting or sustaining an erection and your testosterone levels are low taking this hormone might be helpful.   Therefore any male who suffers form low libido and erectile problems should have his testosterone measured.   If levels are low and here we are talking less than 14nmol/Litre then replacement might help to restore flagging erectile function.   A good dose would be 25-75 mg per day taken in divided doses either in the form of a troche or cream.   Regular surveillance of testosterone levels is mandatory once this treatment is initiated, as well as periodic monitoring of prostate status, via a PSA test and an internal examination, a blood count and cholesterol levels.

In my clinical practice I've treated a number of men and women with low testosterone levels who have appreciated the boost that this hormone has provided to their sexual function both in terms of desire and increased pleasure.

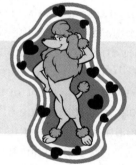

Hormones can help to
unleash sexual power

OESTROGEN AND PROGESTERONE

If testosterone is the libido hormone then oestrogen comes a close second as far as stimulating female sexual desire, arousal and mood is concerned.   Studies have shown that hormone replacement therapy in the form of oestrogen improves sexual desire in postmenopausal women. (5) In the postmenopausal context women who take hormones experience less sexual dysfunction than those who don't. (6) It is oestrogen which ensures that the female genital tract is provided with a good blood supply and adequate lubrication and is primarily responsible for maintaining the structural integrity of vaginal tissue, all necessary ingredients for healthy sexual function. In addition to which Italian sexual dysfunction expert Dr Alessandra Graziottin tells us that oestrogen's unique role is to safeguard female sensuality by preserving all the primary senses including touch, taste, smell, hearing and eyesight. (7) Without sufficient oestrogen Graziottin explains, all female senses will be dulled and deprived of the lubrication, sensitivity and awareness needed to enjoy the completeness of the sexual experience.

Progesterone's position is less clear. The late Dr John Lee who pioneered the importance of this hormone was of the opinion that women need small amounts of progesterone to stimulate sex drive especially in the menopausal context when this hormone is lacking. (8) Dr Graziottin has a different point of view reminding us that there is often an increase in sexual desire premenstrually when progesterone levels are low suggesting that the presence of this hormone puts a damper on sexual function. Female mice without oestrogen aren't provoked into sexual behaviour when stimulated by progesterone and an Australian study has shown that progesterone cream failed to evoke sexual feelings when administered to postmenopausal women over a twelve-week period indicating that aside from possibly inhibiting sexual response this hormone is not critical for female sexual function. (9)

Ironically men need oestrogen almost as much as women. Receptors for this female hormone are located in the brain and the penis with good evidence that arousal, erectile function and even fertility are primed by the presence of this hormone. The male body in its wisdom uses testosterone to make oestrogen via an enzyme called aromatase and it is this traditionally female essence that is interwoven with the male sexual experience. However too much oestrogen can interfere with male sexual activity as the overabundance of this hormone, which often occurs in the overweight male, can switch off testosterone production and might also be harmful to the prostate. Once again hormonal balance defines the nature of optimal sexual function. Both sexes need each other's hormones in just the right proportions for a healthy sex life.

DEHYDROEPIANDROSTERONE (DHEA)

DHEA is a wonderfully bisexual hormone in that it has the ability to either make testosterone or oestrogen in both sexes depending on which hormone is needed. DHEA travels around the body and is used to manufacture oestrogen if that is the hormone that is lacking or testosterone if that's what the body needs. And this happens in both sexes. Women are especially reliant on DHEA. Premenopausally DHEA contributes significantly to female oestrogen and testosterone and after the menopausal transition this hormone is the sole provider for these hormones. Men also use DHEA as a supply source for their testosterone needs so it comes as no surprise when studies reveal that low levels of this hormone leads to sexual problems in both sexes. Men with low DHEA have erectile problems while women who are deficient have libido, arousal and orgasmic difficulties. (10) (11) Replenish DHEA and you can turn sexual misery into orgasmic delight.

Trials performed on both sexes with low DHEA levels show that erectile dysfunction and female sexual disorders can be remedied with DHEA. (12) (13) The real art lies in providing the correct dose of this hormone. Too much DHEA can oversupply the male with oestrogen and inundate the female with testosterone. What I do in my clinic is measure DHEA, testosterone and oestrogen levels in both sexes before and during treatment. This should be done every three months to ensure that the levels of these hormones are maintained in the right zone. To limit the formation of excessive oestrogen in the male context various remedies can be used, both pharmaceutical and natural, to reduce the activity of aromatase, the enzyme that produces oestrogen.

Aromatase inhibitors that reduce oestrogen

- The drug arimidex at a dose of ½ mg twice weekly.
- The antioxidant resveratrol, made from the skins of red grapes, 5mg daily.
- Quercetin, a vitamin-like substance, 500mg three times daily.
- Correcting zinc deficiency and supplementing with zinc chelate 15-30 mg daily.
- Progesterone cream 10-15mg applied at night.
- Chrysin, a type of antioxidant known as a flavonoid, 300mg daily.

Consuming extra soy is another option. You can try a combination of the above as well as maintaining a healthy weight. Although I have a preference for natural remedies my experience with arimidex indicates that this appears to be the most effective option for tempering the excessive accumulation of oestrogen.

Utilizing DHEA in the female context can be less complicated. I have found that starting off with a low dose of 10mg daily or 25mg every second day doesn't usually result in high testosterone levels. Progesterone can also help to lower testosterone when taken together with DHEA.

THYROID HORMONE

As this hormone effects circulation, energy and mood having low levels of thyroid hormone will certainly not have a favourable impact on sexual activity. One review has demonstrated that men with erectile dysfunction can have low thyroid hormone levels and once these have been corrected this problem can be reversed. Ensuring that you are well served by thyroid hormones both by means of blood tests and morning temperature evaluation will provide you with one of the foundations for a healthy sex life.

Hormones are unquestionably amongst the principal players in this exquisitely complex sexual saga. What men also need is a good circulation. Poor blood supply is thought to be one of the determining events that ultimately weakens the muscular function which is so vital for having an erection. (14) (15) Erectile problems are thought to be an early warning signal that other critically important vascular channels such as those which serve the heart might also be compromised. Any man who is struggling in this area needs to have his cholesterol evaluated along with the other measures, which will be detailed in the chapter on hearts and brains, that establish whether his cardiovascular system is in good working order.

To recap, hormones stoke your sexual fires and if the flames are dying for no particular reason then you need to have those powerful chemicals measured. Here are the major hormones that matter.

Hormones that influence male erectile function:

- Testosterone
- Growth hormone
- Thyroid hormone
- DHEA

Hormones that impact female sexual function:

- Oestrogen
- Testosterone
- DHEA

There's even the case of a woman who endured a life-long absence of sexual drive only to have this turned around by the application of dihydrotestosterone, a stronger form of the hormone testosterone, to her external genitalia.

Hormones have the power but there are also natural remedies that have the ability to restore hormonal balance, improve circulation and work in ways similar to that of drugs like viagra to help with sexual difficulties. If you want to boost your body's intrinsic process and augment hormonal function in a subtler fashion then these therapies might be a good place to start. Here are the herbs, vitamins, antioxidants and natural therapies that can be used to manage male and female sexual problems in turn.

Natural remedies for erectile dysfunction:

- Gingko biloba at a dose of two 60mg tablets twice daily.
- The amino acid L-arginine taken in high doses of up to 6 grams daily. This can be reduced when combined with the antioxidant pycnogenol as documented by a study, which has shown that 1.7 grams of L-arginine can revive ailing erectile function when combined with three 40mg pycnogenol tablets. (16)
- The herb Korean red ginseng at a dose of 900mg three times daily has been found to be significantly more effective than placebo when used to treat erectile dysfunction. (17)
- Zinc, especially when there are deficiencies of this nutrient, can increase testosterone levels and renew sexual potency. (18) A good dose would be 30mg daily.
- Butea superba and icariin are two new herbal kids on the block from Thailand, which have been utilised in clinical trials to treat erectile dysfunction. (19) (20) Interestingly icariin's method of action is like that of the viagra-like agents, which inhibit an enzyme called phosphodiesterase E5 thereby allowing blood to enter the penis. This mechanism re-establishes an erectile response.
- Maca, a herb grown around the mountains of Peru, at a daily dose of 1500-3000mg has been shown to increase sexual desire without raising hormonal levels. (21)

- Tribulus terrestris - 250mg of the herb taken three times daily might have aphrodisiac properties by increasing testosterone levels.

Natural remedies for female sexual dysfunction

- Muira puama, a South American herb, and gingko biloba improved a host of parameters assessed over a one-month period in pre and post-menopausal women complaining of low sex drive. (22) This included improvements in libido, frequency of sexual fantasies and sexual intercourse, ability to reach orgasm and intensity of orgasm. The fact that all these developments manifested after only one months worth of treatment constitutes a sensational response.

- Taking 3000mg of vitamin C daily, which is quite a high dose, has been shown to increase intercourse frequency and mood in a group of healthy young adults both female and male. (23) Who said there was no scientific evidence for the use of vitamin C? Then there are the topical treatments such as viacreme and womanzone touted as 'the ultimate female gel' which contain L-arginine and a number of other ingredients designed to boost circulation and enhance sensitivity when applied to the genitals. Clinical trials performed by the originators of womanzone indicate that women who have used these gels experience easier arousal, increased pleasurable sensations and more intense orgasms.

Finally this chapter wouldn't be complete without due consideration being given to two common male problems, premature ejaculation and Peyronie's disease.

PREMATURE EJACULATION

Medications are now replacing psychological and behavioural treatments for this troubling problem and there probably isn't a male on the planet who hasn't been there at some stage of his life. The sad news is that the current crop of treatments such as the antidepressant medications which increase serotonin levels have a significant side-effect profile of their own and topical applications of anaesthetic agents aren't that appealing when these need to be applied in the middle of a passionate love-making session. On the bright side, we now know via animal studies that there is a distinct circuitry of nerves that control ejaculation and so the race is on to devise some form of palatable medication which prevents the poor hapless male from powering to the finish line before the race has started. Until that happens the good old-fashioned squeeze technique still appears to be the most attractive option. And it's natural.

PEYRONIE'S DISEASE

This unfortunate disorder results from fibrous growths at the base of the penis, which can be painful and even lead to curvature of this vital organ making intercourse difficult if not sometimes downright impossible. The marvels of modern surgery have all sorts of wonderful techniques to correct this deformity but for the more patient there is an array of topical treatments to choose from including the application of verapamil, the drug used to treat high blood pressure, the combination of L-arginine and viagra and then there's testosterone and the stronger dihydrotestosterone also used around the area where there is fibrosis. The latter remedy is endorsed by Belgian hormonal expert Thierry Hertoghe.

There is also a study which indicates that acetyl-L-carnitine 1 gram taken orally twice daily has the ability to reduce the curvature of the penis and prevent this process from progressing and another study demonstrating that combining vitamin E 600mg daily with colchicine 1mg twice daily which is a drug usually reserved for the treatment of gout can ease any discomfort and can similarly stop this disorder from getting any worse. (24) (25) If you aren't too keen on having surgery there are a number of natural options you can turn to in order to manage this problem.

There we have it, hormones and an assortment of natural remedies to stimulate, lubricate and regenerate your sexual energy. Unlike viagra and the similar medications these aren't a quick fix. For example testosterone can take a while to alleviate erectile dysfunction. It may not happen overnight but it will happen.

Many of the women with whom I consult during menopause and beyond are having a difficult time of it. Around the menopausal transition and soon thereafter many women appear to gain weight, suffer from low energy, depression, poor sleeping patterns, severe stress and experience difficulties with hot flushes and dry skin. They are struggling to function on a daily basis and they want their health back. Conventional HRT often has side effects and doesn't seem to deal with all these problems in a satisfactory fashion. The question is how do we manage these hormonal challenges in the best possible way?

As I indicated in the beginning of this book my preference is to use a gentler yet effective form of hormone treatment called bio-identical hormone replacement. This is how this treatment works. Oestrogen is found in the body in three major forms: oestradiol, which is manufactured in the premenopausal period and is the strongest form of oestrogen in terms of its stimulatory effects on the female body. Approximately 10% of oestrogen is comprised of oestradiol. Oestrone is made in the postmenopausal period, is less powerful than oestradiol and forms 10% of total oestrogen. Oestriol is the third oestrogen and is by far the weakest component of this trio. This hormone is secreted during pregnancy and occupies the final 80% of circulating oestrogen. Triest meaning three oestrogens is a combination of these three principal oestrogens in the same ratios that are found in the body. This ingenious formulation was devised by Dr Jonathon Wright, an American doctor who sought to provide a remedy which had all the oestrogen-like benefits, while minimising any negative effects that this hormone may have on the body. The idea was to treat hot flushes, balance the emotional state, preserve the integrity of genital tissue and prevent the diseases of ageing such as osteoporosis, heart disease and dementia while avoiding the development of cancer of the breast and the lining of the womb.

The difference between this type of hormone delivery system and conventional hormone treatment is not so much that it is natural, as the patches and gels, which are the mainstays of regular hormone replacement, are derived from soy and wild yam in the same way as these. The cardinal difference lies in the combinations of hormones that are delivered in that the oestrogens are milder than conventional treatments and therefore safer in theory and the dosage can also be modified to suit individual needs based upon hormonal levels. This allows for much more leeway to manoeuvre and adjust dosages whereas with conventional treatment there aren't many sizes from which to choose.

The other primary female hormone is progesterone. Progesterone is the hormone that imparts balance thereby offsetting any detrimental effects that excessive oestrogen stimulation might have on breast tissue or the lining of the uterus. There is also the possibility that this hormone builds stronger bones. Natural progesterone that is incorporated in bio-identical hormone replacement resembles the progesterone found in the female body and is not the same as the synthetic progestin found in conventional hormone replacement. Synthetic progestin found in Provera is structurally slightly different from progesterone and like Premarin is also thought to be responsible for some of the adverse outcomes associated with hormone replacement. including bloating, breast tenderness, weight gain and the increased incidence of heart disease and possibly even breast cancer. (1) (2) (3) (4) (5) (6) (7)

Case studies

Sarah is a 50 year-old executive assistant whose periods had ceased at the age of 48. She was suffering from hot flushes, had aches all over her body and her skin was as dry as the Sahara. Going bald was something only men have to put up with so it was a source of major embarrassment and distress when she started to notice that she was losing her hair. She was also mortified by the accumulation of fat around her abdomen, as she had been a past member of the national basketball team.

I reassured her that once we measured her hormones we would find that there was a lot that we could do to improve her situation. Indeed her hormonal profile revealed that she had low levels of oestrogen and progesterone. Her DHEA and testosterone levels were also under the ideal range and her body was not producing enough thyroid hormone.

Her biochemical picture indicated that she had insulin resistance, which made it difficult for her to lose weight and her liver function demonstrated elevation of her enzymes further compounding her problems. I informed Sarah that we needed to boost her hormones, manage her insulin resistance and improve her liver function and once we did this she would start to see an upswing in her fortunes. She commenced hormone treatment in the form of a troche, which is a lozenge that allows the hormones to dissolve inside the cheek and enter the bloodstream. She also started taking kelp to boost her thyroid function, undertook to reduce her consumption of carbohydrates and fats and to increase her intake of protein and low glycaemic index foods. She was also advised to take a herbal compound to improve her liver function as well as alpha-lipoic acid and chromium to make it easier for her insulin to operate effectively. Hopefully this would help her body to burn fat and lose weight.

The following was her treatment regimen:

- Triest 0.5 mg
- Testosterone 0.25mg
- DHEA 5mg
- Progesterone 50mg
  Taken twice daily-morning and mid afternoon

- Kelp 500mg *twice daily*

- St Mary's thistle *combined with other herbs to improve liver function*

- Alpha lipoic acid 100mg *twice daily*

- Chromium nicotinate 200mcg *three times daily with meals.*

When she returned to see me after three months her hormone levels had improved, her hot flushes were no longer troubling her, the aches occurred far less frequently and she was starting to lose weight. Her skin was no longer dry and she was also extremely pleased to announce that her hair loss was abating. Her repeat blood tests also indicated that her insulin and blood sugar levels were normalising, her thyroid function had improved and her liver enzymes were no longer elevated.

I have reviewed Sarah on a three monthly basis and have repeated her hormone assays on each occasion making sure that her levels remain within optimal limits. She has been overjoyed with her progress as she is rapidly approaching her ideal weight and her hair loss has virtually ceased.

Lee, a 45 year-old high-powered business-woman had to deal with a host of difficulties including repeated bouts of depression, an average of five hours sleep per night and dare I say it overwhelming fatigue. Somehow, as if she had an endless reservoir of energy to tap in to, she managed to keep it all together which included the demands of her job, her husband and her three children. When I saw her, her periods had become irregular and infrequent and she had the hint of an occasional hot flush. I had the sense that the inordinate amount of stress that she was under was propelling her towards the menopause and she was existing on pure adrenaline with hormones in short supply. Her hormonal assays confirmed my suspicions. Her progesterone levels were low which can exacerbate anxiety and sleeplessness. Her DHEA levels were virtually non-existent, a not unusual development in anyone who is extended to the limit.

What we did was institute low dose hormone treatment via progesterone cream at a dose of 20mg applied to the skin at night from days 5-26 of her menstrual cycle, as well as 10mg of DHEA taken daily. The progesterone was designed to make it easier for her to get some quality sleep, which would help to relieve her anxiety and I was hoping that the DHEA would reduce her depression and give her more energy. This regimen really worked a treat as when she returned I was immediately struck by a remarkable transformation. She was sleeping through the night and her depression had lifted. Her daily stresses appeared less overwhelming which provided her with renewed energy. The hot flushes, which were beginning to surface, were no longer present. Her hormonal regimen had thrown her a lifeline and she was incredibly grateful.

I see many women just like Lee who are thrust prematurely into menopause because their ovaries are starting to wind down and their adrenals are labouring to keep up with the pace of their stressful lives. If you've hit your forties, your periods are starting to become irregular, you're feeling moody and depressed for no reason, your muscles are starting to lose their tone, your sex drive is in neutral, your skin is starting to hang and your flab is hard to shift, have your hormones measured. You might find that you have very little DHEA and your supplies of progesterone are also tapering off. I have found that using small amounts of progesterone is all that is needed to deal with anxiety and sleeplessness. What this hormone can also do is to make your cells more responsive to whatever oestrogen you have floating around your bloodstream, which would help to nourish your skin and alleviate hot flushes. DHEA would further replenish oestrogen and also give testosterone a boost, which might make it easier to stay trim, taut and terrific and keep that middle-aged spread at bay.

Hormones can help you stop the menopause blues

The same principles apply when you've passed through the menopause and beyond. If you're not happy with your energy or your health, you've tried conventional HRT and it hasn't worked for you or you just simply want to get your moods and your vitality back on track then you need to have your hormones evaluated. I do this with all my patients, as I believe it's important to establish a baseline and find out where the real deficiencies lie.

Mary faced that kind of predicament. She is a 59 year-old saleslady who had been taking a hormone called tibolone for over a year until she found that she was becoming increasingly bloated and felt that this treatment was making her gain weight. She wanted a form of hormone treatment that wouldn't have these side-effects while at the same time she enjoyed a healthy sex life and certainly didn't want this part of her life to diminish in any way. She'd heard that I prescribed what she understood was a more natural form of HRT and she also wondered whether this type of treatment would help to prevent osteoporosis and Alzheimer's disease as she had a family history of both. All Mary's hormone levels were extremely low which we would expect in a 59 year-old who had ceased hormone treatment.

She started on the following:

- Triest 1mg
- Progesterone 200mg   *½ troche taken twice daily*
- Testosterone 1mg
- DHEA 20 mg

This is the kind of combination that I commence in most of my patients who are lacking in these hormones. You will notice that the amount of hormones in Mary's formulation is greater than that of Sarah. This is because Mary is older and her body wasn't able to provide her with much in the way of hormones at all. How is the dose of each hormone that is included in this troche formulation derived and why the combination? With all the controversy surrounding the relationship between hormone replacement and the development of cancers of the breast and the lining of the womb as well as heart disease, scientists have attempted to derive a replacement dosage that would alleviate all those symptoms troubling women as they go through menopause, go some way to preventing any diseases happening further down the track while at the some time minimizing any risks of excessive hormonal stimulation.

Recent research indicates that this might just be on the cards with a number of studies showing that lower doses of conjugated equine oestrogen or premarin and medroxyprogesterone acetate or provera at 0.3mg and 1.5 mg per day respectively are sufficient to relieve hot flushes, protect the lining of the uterus, make sure that vaginal tissue stays healthy and increase bone mineral density. (8) (9)) Triest 1mg equates to premarin 0.3mg which makes this an ideal formulation to manage the problems associated with menopause while also offering the potential to preserve strong, healthy bones and to prevent heart disease and Alzheimer's.   Once you commence this form of hormone replacement it's a good idea to have your hormones measured by means of a blood test to ensure that you are receiving the amount of hormones that is protective and not harmful. An ideal time to do this is 4-5 hours after you've taken your hormones in the morning. The optimal level of oestrogen that is thought to prevent heart disease, safeguard your mental powers while not being harmful to your breasts lies between 150-250pmol/Litre or 60-100pg/ml. It would be to your advantage to have this evaluation every 3-6 months just to make sure that you are receiving healthy amounts of oestrogen. Naturally you also want the hormones you are taking to alleviate any uncomfortable symptoms you might have had and more importantly to make you feel good.

The beauty of triest is that you don't have to be exposed to excessive levels of individual hormones. Balance and the appropriate quantity of each hormone is the key. The three oestrogens in triest provide you with the benefits of each oestrogen in turn without overstepping the limits of these hormones. Some women might even find that this form of HRT is too stimulating for them. Swollen breasts, weight gain and the other problems resulting from excessive oestrogen stimulation described in chapter two can be managed by utilising oestriol, the much weaker oestrogen, on its own.

Oestriol has been shown to be effective for treating hot flushes, insomnia, headaches and even depression and poor memory. Oestriol can also be incorporated to preserve healthy vaginal tissue and to prevent those troublesome bladder infections that occur with oestrogen deficiency. This can be achieved by applying this hormone topically to the genital area and what this does is to reduce vaginal pH and increase the growth of protective bacteria called lactobacilli, which neutralizes the presence of any harmful germs. Oestriol can thicken the skin, reduce dryness and has been used to treat wrinkles.

I had one patient who was approaching the menopause and she was suffering from severe migraines especially around her periods. All she needed to do was to apply some oestriol cream to her skin during the second half of the cycle and during her period, when her body produced less oestrogen and this had the desired result of putting an end to her migraines. Some of my patients have used oestriol to restore moisture and texture to their dry skins. Oestriol can lower cholesterol and prevent osteoporosis when taken in high doses. The initial dose of oestriol would be 4-8mg either via the troche or the skin. On the other hand, there might be other women who find the dose of triest to be too mild to relieve their symptoms and then we have to either increase the dose or to change to oestradiol the stronger oestrogen on its own without the diluting effect of the two weaker oestrogens. Initially a low dose in the order of ¼ -½ mg of oestradiol either by means of a troche or applied to the skin would be used. There is no set formula. Each woman has a unique hormonal chemistry and this has to be catered for by means of trial and error.

In addition to its protective effects on the lining of the uterus and its potential to ward off breast cancer progesterone is included because of its calming effects on the nervous system and the possibility that it might contribute to building strong bones. This hormone can be especially useful in the time leading up to the menopause, also known as the perimenopausal period, for managing anxiety and sleeplessness and when taken at night can work really well to calm the nervous system and promote a good night's rest. Hot flushes can also be managed effectively with progesterone as it is thought that this hormone potentiates the action of oestrogen, which might be diminishing during this time.

During the perimenopause a therapeutic dose would be 20mg applied to the skin from days 8-20, which increases to 40mg for days 21-28.

If you're using the combination of hormones that I've described after the menopause, which includes oestrogen, then you need a certain amount of progesterone to protect the lining of your uterus from the effects of excessive oestrogen stimulation. The same blood test that is performed to establish that you have effective levels of oestrogen can also be used to measure progesterone. An ideal level of progesterone that would achieve this kind of protection would be 5-10nmol/Litre or 2-5ng/mL. To achieve this kind of protection you need to take at least 40-60mg of progesterone cream or 200-400mg of the troche. There are some experts who claim that to achieve a protective level of progesterone you need at least 100mg of this hormone applied to your skin, which is much higher than the amount I'm suggesting. I have found that too much progesterone can make you drowsy and depressed not to mention the fact that excessive replacement with this hormone can worsen insulin resistance.

What you need to do to establish whether you are receiving protective quantities of progesterone is to have regular ultrasound checks of the lining of your uterus. If your lining is becoming excessively thickened this means you are either receiving too much oestrogen or not enough progesterone and you will have to adjust your dosage accordingly.

Testosterone and DHEA are included in the troche as they have the potential to alleviate fatigue, stir the sexual fires that might be smoldering and help with that enduring weight loss problem. Testosterone stimulates muscle growth and aside from giving you a better shape, muscle burns fat. There is also evidence that both these hormones increase bone mineralisation and bone strength. (10) DHEA has the ability to boost the immune system, improve memory, alleviate depression and, like progesterone, might be protective against breast cancer. Your blood test and the way you respond to these hormones will tell you whether they suit you or not. An ideal level of testosterone that boosts your sexual energy and keeps your muscles in good shape while not making you manly in any way would be 2-3nmol/Litre. It's important not to overshoot the mark with testosterone as too much of this hormone can worsen insulin resistance making it even more difficult for you to lose weight. A healthy amount of DHEA as evaluated by your blood test would be 5-10umol/Litre.

You can take hormones either in the form of troches, which you put in your mouth, or cream, which you apply to your skin. Each has their advantages and their drawbacks. Some of my patients find that the troches are more effective and more powerful. Troche formulations are usually easy to take and they can have favourable effects on your cholesterol levels by increasing HDL and lowering LDL. However when you allow the hormones to melt inside your cheek it is virtually impossible not to swallow some of these chemicals. From your digestive system they travel to your liver where they have the potential to increase the carrier protein called sex hormone binding globulin as well as clotting factors that interfere with the normal flow of your blood. Having more sex hormone binding globulin can reduce the potency of the hormones that you are taking. I have found that a healthy functioning liver does not make excessive amounts of sex hormone binding globulin and if you want to improve your liver function you can take herbal tonics such as st mary's thistle. Limiting your consumption of soy products also lessens sex hormone binding globulin.

Fibrinogen is one of the clotting factors that you can have measured before you commence this treatment. You can monitor this protein to ensure that levels remain within reasonable limits. Vitamin E, the B vitamins, folic acid, omega-3 fatty acids found in fish and flaxseed oil and the herb gingko biloba keep your blood flowing nice and smoothly. This limits any harm that extra clotting factors might cause. A way out of this dilemma is to insert the troche under the tongue rather than inside your cheek. This will reduce the amount of troche that you swallow as most of it will be absorbed under your tongue and this will have less of an effect on the liver and sex hormone binding globulin.

Another option is to utilize the creams instead of the troches, which do not travel to your liver and therefore will not raise sex hormone binding globulin or stimulate the manufacture of clotting factors.

Some women prefer to utilise HRT on a continuous basis as it reduces the occurrence of any annoying menstrual bleeding and stopping their hormones reawakens all their symptoms with a vengeance. However, if you find that you need to constantly increase your dose then having a few days break at the end of each month might give your hormone receptors a certain amount of respite. This might reduce the necessity to repeatedly adjust your treatment. My preference is to suggest that you do have 3-5 days without taking hormones at the end of every month. Your body might become used to this after a while so that the recurring menstrual type bleeding ceases. Hormones function by way of activating receptors, which are found on the membranes of your cells and allowing your receptors some hormone-free time means that they will be primed and ready when you recommence your treatment at the beginning of each month.

Once you have commenced hormone replacement therapy it would also be a good idea to have your cholesterol levels as well as lipoprotein (a), another form of fat, which can block your blood vessels, checked regularly. It is worthwhile ensuring that these are not affected in any adverse way.

For those who want to explore the natural alternatives for managing the symptoms of menopause before they embrace hormone treatments there are a number of remedies from which to choose.

Treating hot flushes and night sweats with natural alternatives

- Avoid spicy foods and limit caffeine and alcohol.
- Of all the herbal remedies black cohosh is the most effective. You can take up to two tablets of a proprietary product called remifenin twice daily. The herb red clover has been found to have a positive effect in some trials but others have been less confirmatory. (11)(12)
- Consuming extra soy can also reduce hot flushes at least in the short-term although the effect might wear off after a while. At a recent health symposium one of the members of the audience asked me how much soy was necessary to treat hot flushes and I really couldn't give her an exact answer. After reading an extensive review, which documented all the trials utilising soy I discovered that ½ litre of soy milk per day, the equivalent of 30-60 grams of soy protein, is sufficient. There has been a lot of negative hype surrounding soy suggesting that the consumption of this substance does us more harm than good by obstructing normal thyroid function and hampering the absorption of the nutrients we need from our bowel. In fact most of the research is positive indicating that soy does not compromise thyroid function, has beneficial effects on cholesterol levels as well as bone density, assists insulin function making it easier for you to lose weight, improves memory and might be protective against the development of breast cancer.

(13)(14)(15)(16)(17)(18)

If these measures are ineffective then you might have to consider some form of hormone treatment, which is without question the most effective means for dealing with the symptoms of menopause and preventing the diseases of ageing with heart disease, dementia and osteoporosis being high on the list of priorities. We will be dealing with heart disease and dementia in an upcoming chapter, which leaves the spotlight shining brightly on osteoporosis. This is a condition which I suggest you go all out to prevent. Like heart disease, osteoporosis is a silent killer. Your bones won't tell you they are crumbling until you sustain that crippling fracture which could lead to a miserable existence filled with incapacity and helplessness. In Australia the lifetime risk of sustaining an osteoporotic fracture after the age of 50 is 42% for women and 27% for men. Astoundingly 20,000 hip fractures, which can lead to permanent immobilisation, are sustained annually in Australia. These are the steps you can take to promote strong and sturdy bones.

PREVENTING OSTEOPOROSIS

To begin with you need to find out whether you have any predisposing factors for developing this condition.

Risk factors

- Being a female. Bone loss starts earlier in women but men start to catch up when they reach the age of 70
- Being postmenopausal
- Being thin
- A family history of osteoporosis and fractures

- Inactivity
- Poor calcium absorption. The ability to absorb calcium decreases with ageing
- Cigarette smoking
- Excessive alcohol consumption
- Overproduction of thyroid hormone
- Long-standing liver and kidney disease
- Inflammation
- Increased free radical levels
- Reduced antioxidant protection
- Elevated homocysteine levels

It might seem politically incorrect to identify the female sex and the postmenopausal years as the prime factors that lead to osteoporosis but this is an unfortunate reality. This is why some form of interventional strategy is so vital. You might be wondering how some of these factors such as inflammation, free radicals and homocysteine relate to the development of osteoporosis.

There is a growing body of research which suggests that heart disease, Alzheimer's dementia and osteoporosis, all predominantly diseases that escalate with ageing, are caused by similar phenomena. Inflammation occurs when the immune system becomes overactive while homocysteine is a protein that accumulates in your body when you have insufficient vitamin B12 and folic acid.

Both inflammation and homocysteine can stir up all sorts of mischief when they are not dealt with appropriately by your body. If these are unchecked they can promote osteoporosis. Fascinatingly what seems to be the most powerful weapon for nullifying the destructive effects that excessive levels of inflammation, free radical stress and homocysteine can have on the female body is none other than oestrogen, the primary female hormone. Oestrogen has massive anti-inflammatory and antioxidant potential and it is this hormone that might be the key to preventing heart disease, dementia and osteoporosis. Before we proceed to discuss hormone treatment let's explore how you can minimise the above risks and elaborate all those steps you can take to enhance your bone health.

THE OPTIMAL DIET

Protein and calcium are the two core nutrients which your body uses to maintain healthy bone tissue. You need just the right amounts of each of these. Excessive protein consumption especially that which is derived from animal sources can make your blood acidic and this can leach calcium away from your bones. Too much red meat might even make your bones fragile as demonstrated by animal studies. (19) One of the long-term dangers of the high protein diet is the possibility that overexposure to large amounts of protein in the face of disproportionately low levels of calcium can lead to loss of bone. 1gram per kilogram of bodyweight per day would be a reasonable amount of protein. Too much salt will also see to it that your body loses extra calcium in your urine. Eating at least five serves of fruit and vegetables a day especially those of the leafy green variety will provide you with nutrients like magnesium, vitamin C, vitamin K and potassium which combine with protein and calcium to preserve strong bones.

CALCIUM

Calcium is a vital bone nutrient. Of that there is no doubt. Just how much calcium we do need is a real bone of contention. The recommended daily requirement for calcium is 1000mg per day and this increases to 1200mg after the age of fifty. From the age of forty women lose bone at an annual rate of 0.5-1% and without sufficient calcium this doubles to 2%. Experts are at pains to tell us that we aren't getting enough calcium from our daily diet and this is understandable when you realise that you have to consume at least 1 litre of milk per day to achieve your recommended rations of 1200mg. This is no easy task. Obtaining adequate amounts of calcium becomes even more difficult with ageing as our digestive systems become less efficient at extracting the essential nutrients that our bodies need from the foods we eat.

How can you tell whether you are getting enough calcium from your diet and whether your body needs calcium? Muscle cramps, irritability and insomnia would suggest that you might have a calcium deficiency. As calcium is such a critical nutrient and is used to control your heartbeat and to regulate your nervous system your body will see to it that you have enough calcium to fulfill these functions by extracting this nutrient from your bones. Therefore the calcium running around in your blood stream will always be the amount your heart and your nervous system needs which means that you might have to be significantly deficient before you develop cramps and an irritable nervous system. Blood tests measuring calcium levels won't help you much either as these will mostly be normal for the reasons already stated.

Tests that can tell you whether you are low in calcium include a bone density test and a parathyroid assay otherwise known as a PTH blood test. PTH is secreted by the parathyroid glands, which sit on top of your thyroid gland, as you would expect and when your calcium levels go down, more PTH will be produced to improve your calcium status. Hence if your PTH levels are starting to climb then you know that you are running into a calcium deficiency problem.

If you are low in calcium there are certain steps you need to take. Firstly you need to ensure that your digestive system is in good shape and that you are absorbing all the calcium you can from the foods you consume. A gluten intolerance can often compromise your digestive capacity and this can be ruled out by a simple blood test, which measures gliadin antibodies. Then you need to find out whether you are getting enough calcium in your diet. Once again this raises a thorny issue and that is the ongoing dispute concerning the best food source of calcium. Supporters of dairy including the dairy board in Australia naturally would provide you with a mountain of evidence which details the connection between high levels of calcium obtained from dairy products and a reduction in fracture rates. They will also tell you that milk provides the most bio-available source of calcium and that you have to gobble down a ton of broccoli to obtain the same amount of calcium from a half a cup of milk.

All of this is true. You do need to consume a whole lot more of your highly nutritious green vegetables to obtain reasonable amounts of calcium. However two dessertspoons of tahini, which is sesame seed spread, will supply you with 1000mg of calcium which is just about all you need to satisfy your daily rations. A handful of almonds and Brazil nuts together with a substantial serve of broccoli, parsley and cauliflower will furnish you with ½ your daily calcium needs and if you add some fortified soymilk then you're just about home and dry. Other good sources of calcium would be small fish like sardines including the bones and hummus otherwise known as chickpea spread.

To square the ledger with dairy products I have to admit that I have a personal bias against this food source. There is evidence linking dairy consumption with a number of diseases including diabetes mellitus, prostate and breast cancer as well as multiple sclerosis. Then there is the rather surprising news that those countries where dairy is highly popular also have increased rates of osteoporosis. To be fair to those who love dairy and want to obtain their calcium from this source, low fat dairy products combined with fruit and vegetables can lower blood pressure and dairy on its own can be used to facilitate weight loss by improving insulin function. The calcium in dairy has been associated with a reduced risk for developing strokes and bowel cancer clearly showing that this substance has benefits.

If you are struggling to meet your daily calcium requirements, your bone density is sub-optimal and you have some of the risk factors for osteoporosis then you might need calcium supplements. These can be found in carbonate or citrate form or you can incorporate the calcium obtained from bonemeal, which is known as microcrystalline hydroxyapatite. A reasonable dose would be 300-500mg daily. Calcium citrate at a dose of 1000-1600mg daily has been shown to substantially reduce bone loss by a healthy 50% with continuous supplementation after menopause resulting in a 50% reduction in fracture rates. This is compared with those women who have not had the benefit of extra calcium. Calcium carbonate would have a similar dosage. Calcium carbonate is absorbed best with meals whereas the citrate form can be taken on an empty stomach and is more easily absorbed in older women who are producing less stomach acid.

For those hapless souls who have already sustained a fracture another form of calcium known as calcium orotate at a dose of 600mg daily can speed up the healing process. One of the nutrients that partners calcium to look after your bones is another mineral that we don't always get enough of in our daily diets and that is magnesium.

MAGNESIUM

As green vegetables and nuts are the major sources of magnesium chances are that you might be hard put to attain your daily quota of this important nutrient. Like calcium magnesium helps to boost bone density and even makes bones more flexible and less brittle which reduces the possibility of developing fractures. Magnesium improves calcium absorption and regulates the transport of this nutrient around the body. Magnesium can also fight inflammation thought to be one of the major causes of osteoporosis with a recent clinical trial showing that rats low in magnesium suffer bone loss due to the activation of pro-inflammatory cells, which increase the activity of osteoclasts, cells responsible for bone resorption or breakdown.

Anxiety, cramps in the calves, twitching eyelids, depression and poor sleep habits raise the possibility that you might be low in magnesium. Blood tests aren't that good at identifying magnesium deficiency and it's probably a good idea to add magnesium to your calcium supplement as these two work hand in glove, 250-400mg of magnesium would be a reasonable dose. Magnesium also assists vitamin D, another nutrient that has a significant impact on bone health.

VITAMIN D

This nutrient is available to you via one of nature's most primitive and powerful forces, the sun. All you have to do is to make sure that you get 5-15 minutes of sunlight 4-6 times per week to expose your skin to all the vitamin D that you need. From your skin vitamin D travels to your liver and then on to your kidneys in order to be potentised so that it can assist with the maintenance of healthy calcium levels and the mineralization of your bones. Vitamin D can also be obtained from fatty fish such as mackerel and herring as well as fortified margarine. Of all the nutrients that have been examined in clinical trials with respect to reducing fracture risk calcium and vitamin D are considered to be the most important for preventing osteoporosis.

There is even some evidence that vitamin D deficiency might increase the risk for developing colon, breast, and prostate cancer and there are trials which suggest that this nutrient can play a part in the treatment regimen for these cancers.

VITAMIN K

Vitamin K is not commonly recognised for its bone boosting properties as this vitamin is usually employed to help you stop bleeding when you cut yourself. However there is some indication that this nutrient also looks after your bones. Once more the green vegetables would be your major supply source with broccoli, spinach, cabbage and kelp providing you with ample amounts of vitamin K. I often hear people complain that they don't enjoy eating green vegetables because they aren't very flavoursome. One method that you can employ to enhance their palatability is to add foods like tahini or hummus or other dips and sauces, which are nutritious in their own right and also make these a real treat to eat.

SOY

Asian women have been using this substance through the ages to improve their health and for good reason. Soy does have the ability to improve bone density and prevent bone breakdown with one proviso. While Asian women need less soy for their bones western women need at least 40g of soy protein to benefit from consuming this nutrient. This means that you have to drink more than a litre of soymilk and eat more than 200g of tempeh per day if you're relying on soy to look after your bones. On the bright side for those who enjoy their soy studies show that the isoflavones found in soy have anti-

inflammatory effects and since inflammation can damage
your bones this should spur you on while you're tucking into
your soy delight.

THE ANTIOXIDANTS

Since excessive levels of free radicals are thought to be
public enemy number one and these are also now being viewed
as the driving force behind the development of osteoporosis it
would be extremely advantageous to understand how these
chemicals operate so that their damaging effects can be
limited. What free radicals do is incite cytokines, those nasty
inflammatory cells that are part of the immune system and
together these pesky critters stimulate the activity of
osteoclasts, the cells that resorb bone, which leads to the
breakdown of your bones. Antioxidants inhibit this process,
which in turn prevents bone loss.

The question is: are there studies out there, which show
that taking antioxidants actually makes bones less vulnerable
and more resilient? Although the human trials have yet to be
performed, there are animal experiments revealing that
antioxidants such as vitamin C and N-acetyl cysteine
effectively abolish bone loss by switching off osteoclasts and
neutralising cytokines. (20) Older women who suffer from
osteoporosis also have markedly decreased antioxidant
defences making their bones less resistant to the demolishing
effects of free radicals. Are these studies enough to justify
antioxidant supplementation? Would it be wise equipping
yourself with added protection against osteoporosis without
substantial scientific confirmation that this is the right thing to
do? Despite the fact that we obviously need more evidence
I'm going to suggest that this would definitely be a wise
choice. 500-1000mg of vitamin C combined with 200-400i.u.
of vitamin E together with 100-200mg of alpha-lipoic acid,

which regenerates these antioxidants once they've done their job, would provide you with a powerful team to defend yourself against an overabundance of free radicals.

VITAMIN B12

This is not a nutrient that you would commonly associate with bone health yet vitamin B12 more often viewed as a learning and memory tonic and a depression and dementia preventive is more that a bit player in this drama. Along with folic acid vitamin B12 suppresses homocysteine, that toxic protein which not only instigates heart disease and cognitive decline but is also thought to set osteoporosis in motion. Many of the folk that I investigate in my clinic have low vitamin B12 levels on their blood tests and this is especially true of vegetarians and the older patients. As studies show that osteoporosis and low vitamin B12 status run in tandem this is one nutrient you really don't want to go without.

THE OTHER NUTRIENTS

Nutrients such as manganese (15-30 mg per day), boron (3-5mg per day), zinc (15-30 mg per day) and copper (13 mg per day) might also be helpful and it would probably be a reasonable proposition to include these in your regimen.

Strontium ranelate is another novel nutrient, not yet available in Australia, that has been shown to boost bone mineral density and reduce fracture rates.

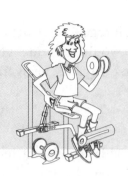

Exercise prevents
your bones from
crumbling

EXERCISE

Regular exercise benefits your bones but more importantly it's the type of exercise that is critical. Going for a brisk walk or jogging is good but it's weight training with increasing levels of resistance that's also going to make a crucial difference.   Stronger muscles build stronger bones. Professor Maria Singh, an exercise and sport science expert from the University of New South Wales in Sydney, emphasises that 2-3 days per week of weight lifting with progressive increments in intensity augments bone density. (21) What you need to do is find a personal trainer who can help you initiate a weight training and aerobic exercise programme and then you should have this plan regularly upgraded so that your weights are increased in accordance with your capabilities. However, there is a limit to the advantages that can be gained from resistance training and an aerobic workout. The more substantial improvements in bone strength are derived from hormone replacement therapy.

THE HORMONES

Even if you had the best diet in the world, you were exercising regularly, getting your fair share of sunlight and taking those nutrients that I've suggested to optimise your bone health you might not be doing all you can to look after your bones. Taking hormones for the long haul might just be the way to ensuring that your bones don't get weaker as you get older. You start to lose bone mass in the premenopausal years and this escalates dramatically once you go through the menopausal transition. It just so happens that this decline in bone mass coincides with a loss of oestrogen once your ovaries start to wind down. (22) After this rapid bone loss your body continues to lose healthy bone but this time at a much more gradual pace. It is thought that this slow yet steady decrease in bone mineralization is also tied in with dwindling supplies of oestrogen. Remember we said that inflammation and free radical excess are major contributors to the erosion of healthy bone and that these destructive processes drive osteoporosis. Guess what? After menopause, when your body is bathed in much less oestrogen, inflammation and free radicals increase significantly. (23) It's therefore not surprising that without oestrogen around to protect you, you are at the mercy of these destructive elements, which have a field day chomping away at your healthy bones.

Aside from oestrogen, progesterone (the other major female hormone) has been shown to have anti-inflammatory properties and there is some evidence that this hormone boosts bone density. Testosterone also has bone-building effects and DHEA has been shown to improve bone mineralization. The same combination of hormones that I described earlier can also be used to nullify any negative factors which may be gaining momentum in your body such as inflammation, the accumulation of free radicals, elevated homocysteine levels and the poor absorption of nutrients. This formulation can be used to see to it that your bones are protected throughout your life.

> ## To refresh your memory here is the formulation again taken in the form of a troche twice daily.
>
> Take ½ troche morning and mid-afternoon or early evening
>
> - Triest 1mg
> - Progesterone 200 mg
> - Testosterone 1mg
> - DHEA 20 mg

It has to be said that triest only contains a small amount of oestradiol, the strongest oestrogen that has the most influential effect on your bones.   For some of you this combination of oestrogens might not be the right strength of hormones particularly if the tests, which evaluate your bone strength, indicate that your bones aren't in good shape. Triest might have to be replaced by the more potent oestrogen in the form of oestradiol if testing indicates that your bone mineral density is diminishing.   If you are taking hormones and these are having a positive effect on your bones then you should continue with this treatment for the long-term. Once you stop taking hormones your risk of developing a fracture is as high as those women who have never used hormone replacement.

If you have a family history of fractures related to osteoporosis and you are a thin person who has gone through early menopause, which is before the age of 48-52, and you register in the affirmative for any of the other risk factors mentioned at the beginning of this section, then you need to consider all the options available to you for safeguarding your bones. This is why you need to have those tests, which will tell you how well your bones are doing.

THE TESTS

BONE MINERAL DENSITY

This is a test which quantifies your bone mineral content in certain strategic areas on your skeleton, such as your hips and your lower back by means of a DEXA scan (a type of X-ray) and then compares this with the average score of a group of young people to see whether your scores differ significantly from the mean. According to the World Health Organisation a score that is more than 2 standard deviations lower than the young average constitutes substantial osteoporosis and is associated with an increased risk of developing fractures. Australian experts recommend treatment for a score this low. There are other tests, which will also provide you with useful information with regard to the status of your bones.

URINE RESORPTION MARKERS

Like the other parts of your body your bones are constantly being remodeled with old bone being replaced by new tissue. Cells that are responsible for bone growth are called osteoblasts while osteoclasts stimulate bone resorption or the breakdown of bone. If resorption were to exceed the capacity of your bones to refashion themselves then you would be entering a state of bone loss, which can be rather substantial around the menopausal period. When this occurs collagen, an essential part of bone, undergoes degradation and substances like deoxypyridinoline and N-telopeptides, the breakdown products of collagen, will be found in excessive amounts in your urine. Analysis of a morning urine specimen will indicate whether abnormally high levels of these substances are present. If this is the case then your bones are breaking down more rapidly than they are being remodeled, and just as you would with a low bone mineral density an action plan needs to be instituted. If you are reluctant to undergo an X-ray, this test can be used instead of a DEXA scan to inform you as to how strong your bones are.

THE OTHER TESTS

To give yourself every chance of being proactive with regard to preventing osteoporosis it would be wise to undergo all those tests, which identify all your risk factors as well as a bone mineral density and/or a urine deoxypyridinoline evaluation.

Here are all those factors as listed at the beginning of this segment and the relevant investigations:

- **Vitamin B12 -**
  a blood test
- **Inflammation-**
  a blood test, which measures highly sensitive C-reactive protein or HS-CRP
- **Homocysteine -**
  a blood test
- **Liver function -**
  a blood test, which will tell you whether you are suffering from inflammation of the liver. The liver potentiates vitamin D
- **Excessive free radical levels -**
  a biological terrain assessment (BTA)test or a urine test, which quantifies a metabolite called 8-hydroxy-2-deoxyguanosine. This will be described in more detail in the final chapter.

- **Parathyroid hormone assay -**
  a blood test. Elevated levels indicate that your calcium supplies are decreasing
- **Vitamin D -**
  a blood test, which evaluates 25OH Vitamin D status

For those who are interested in the Rolls Royce of health assessments and are concerned about optimising their well-being and preventing the diseases of ageing, the final chapter will present you with a detailed protocol for achieving these objectives.

Prescription for bone health

- A healthy diet including adequate amounts of protein, fruit and vegetables
- Regular aerobic exercise and weight training
- At least 15 minutes of sunlight 4-6 times weekly which provides essential vitamin D
- Oestrogen
- Progesterone
- Testosterone
- DHEA
- Calcium
- Magnesium
- Vitamin B12, vitamin C, vitamin E, vitamin K, zinc, manganese, boron, copper and alpha-lipoic acid are minor players but these also contribute to the health of your bones.

MALE MENOPAUSE

Sam, 46, Henry 54, and Lucas 72 had a lot in common. They weren't happy with their energy levels, their sexual capacities had dwindled and their once lean torsos were being reshaped by ever increasing layers of flab. They also shared another widespread handicap, low testosterone levels. Once this problem was addressed and testosterone levels were boosted all three noticed improvements in their energy, their sexual function and their body shape. Their physiques started to shed some of that unwanted fat and regain some of the muscular definition they had lost. Their sex drive and the quality of their erections improved substantially.

Sam, Henry and Lucas represent a typical cross-section of the male patients that I treat regularly in my practice. There are many men out there who are fighting an uphill battle because they don't have enough testosterone and they aren't getting help. I, like many other doctors, believe that there are a large group of men who do go through menopause or andropause as it is termed. They don't have the energy, the endurance, the muscular definition or the strength they used to enjoy.

If your vitality is not what it used to be and you have lost your sexual passion and your lust for life and love then you might have become what is endearingly termed 'the grumpy old man.' If you are a sad, unmotivated grouch who is struggling to keep up and you are gaining fat and losing muscle, there might be a very simple reason for this. All of these events might be due to one elementary and very correctable phenomenon - low testosterone levels. If you suffer from fatigue, diminishing sexual function, you're fighting the battle of the bulge and your mental powers are fading then you need to have your testosterone levels checked. If they are on the low side of normal and here I'm talking in the ballpark of 8-15 mmol/L then testosterone could be responsible for these problems. Enhancing testosterone might be just the tonic you need to boost your energy, improve your mood and augment your sexual vitality.

A healthy kick-off dosage of testosterone would be 25-50mg in divided doses daily taken in either the form of a troche or cream, which should increase the blood level of testosterone to 20-30mmol/Litre. Regular 3-6 monthly checks of the prostate via a PSA blood test and an internal examination are mandatory. Monitoring cholesterol and blood counts to make sure these aren't affected in an adverse way is also important. How to protect your prostate will be discussed in the next chapter.

MEN AND OSTEOPOROSIS

Osteoporosis is a problem that threatens men as they get older almost as much as it does women. Hormones once again are the primary agents that lead to bone loss but the male experience is a little different. Because the male sex don't experience the same dramatic decline in hormone production men have to cope with a gradual loss of bone, which coincides with the progressive loss of testosterone. Ironically it is the female hormone oestrogen that has a major impact on preserving healthy male bone. Men make oestrogen from testosterone and as their supplies of this hormone start to dry up less becomes available to manufacture female hormones. Men need between 90-110 pmol/L of oestrogen to maintain good bone density. Growth hormone also chips in to look after male bones. Therefore men need reasonable amounts of testosterone, oestrogen and growth hormone to look after their bones and for most these are the hormones which are in short supply with ageing.

Although the lead roles reveal some minor variations the script is essentially remarkably similar to the female experience. All the risk factors such as inflammation, free radical excess, elevated homocysteine levels, calcium and magnesium deficiencies and the others mentioned earlier are exactly the same. Men need the same nutrients and should have the same tests and take the same precautions that women do to safeguard bone health. Men should read the preceding segment for women to see how this can be achieved. If testosterone and growth hormone levels are low then these might need to be replenished to sustain healthy bone mineral density.

CHAPTER 7

Fighting Cancer: Prevention and Treatment

I first saw Jane (61) when her bowel cancer had spread to her liver. The medical treatment that she was receiving wasn't able to contain her disease and having exhausted all his options her oncologist decided that she had nothing to lose by exploring some alternative avenues so he referred her to me. I don't think he held out much hope and quite frankly neither did I. But Jane certainly wasn't ready to concede defeat and I wasn't about to tell her that her chances were slim. I didn't possess any guaranteed cure but had some ideas about how we could proceed. We improved her eating habits by removing some of the fat and sugar from her diet and she commenced a combination of remedies including melatonin, the herbal medicines astragalus and Tahitian noni juice to boost her immune system and fight the cancer, as well as a mixture of acidophilus and bifidus to replenish the beneficial germs of her bowel.

Much to my delight and her amazement after two months of this rather simple regimen she started to notice marked improvements. Not only did she feel better but also her blood test, which monitored her liver function, indicated that her enzymes, which were markedly elevated, had started to normalise. Not expecting this dramatic change in her fortunes her oncologist was speechless. A further two months passed and this time her liver panel was totally normal. With tremendous optimism she went for a scan and much to our surprise the cancer that had spread to her liver had completely disappeared. What had happened was beyond my wildest expectations. Within six months she appeared to be free of the disease that had ravaged her body and virtually claimed her life. Jane thought it would be a good idea to continue with her treatment notwithstanding the results of her tests and the last time I saw her she had returned to my clinic with a marked spring in her step to top up the supplies of her medicines. As far as I know she is living a healthy and productive life.

Cancer has to be the toughest health challenge that anyone could face. What you can do though is fight with every weapon at your disposal and this is where you can incorporate hormones, vitamins, herbal medicines, dietary interventions and other supplementary strategies when you enter the battle. You don't develop cancer overnight. The story all revolves around your DNA. This is the core of your genetic hard-drive that programmes the structure and function of your cells, which are constantly replicating. Because your DNA is exposed to a constant barrage of insults, a certain amount of damage erodes the configuration of this vital structure.

In the normal course of events your in-built cellular defences are able to repair any abnormal DNA so that your cells multiply without any blemishes. It is only when this repair mechanism becomes faulty that defective DNA establishes itself leading to the proliferation of those cells, which culminates in the development of cancer. The good news is there is a test that is becoming increasingly more available called the micronucleus assay, which measures DNA damage and is able to inform you how your DNA repair mechanisms are shaping up. A high score would indicate that flawed DNA is setting up shop and that you would need to take the necessary steps to correct this to prevent cancer cells from multiplying. It can take a good 10-20 years for these cells to accumulate before that seemingly innocuous little lump that is a cancer gets your attention and during this time there is a lot you can do to prevent these events from taking hold in your body.

You need to minimise those factors that threaten the integrity of your DNA and these are comprised of many of your familiar foes including free radical excess, hormonal imbalance, elevated homocysteine, inflammation and the debut of some new players. The truth is we all have cancer cells that are trying to gain a foothold in our bodies. But we are able to defend ourselves against these cells and effectively neutralize them. However if your natural defence mechanisms are overwhelmed by excessive amounts of free radicals, inflammation and homocysteine and you also suffer from hormonal imbalance then these cancer cells might be able to thrive without your awareness. This is why you have to have the tests which evaluate whether you have these primary instigators and then you need to deal effectively with them before it is too late. That is before your attention is drawn to the lump I've just mentioned. The major cancers are typical examples of the evolution of this drama both with regard to prevention and treatment.

BREAST CANCER

In the year 2000 over 11,000 new cases of breast cancer were diagnosed in Australia. Any woman has a 1 in 11 chance of developing this form of cancer in her lifetime and the odds increase with age.

RISK FACTORS FOR BREAST CANCER

THE HORMONES

OESTROGEN

I think it's fair to say that women are much more complicated than the males of the species and it probably has a lot to do with the hormone oestrogen. All the evidence seems to suggest that having too much of this hormone may be detrimental as far as breast cancer is concerned. Early menarche, late menopause, becoming pregnant late in life and having few pregnancies, elevated bone mineral density and dense breasts on mammography - all of which are associated with increased exposure to oestrogen - heighten the possibility of developing cancer. In fact excessive oestrogen in the bloodstream does raise the odds which is why it would be a good idea to have your oestrogen levels constantly monitored if you are taking hormones, with healthy supplies of this hormone lying between 150-250pmol/L once you are postmenopausal. (1)

The real burning question is whether hormone replacement actually places you in danger and here the answer is probably not. There is a slightly increased risk of developing breast cancer with different forms of hormone replacement therapy. However it is possible that the culprit might be the synthetic progestins, which are structurally different from natural progesterone rather than the oestrogen component of these formulations. With regard to the much publicised negative findings in the Women's Health Initiative trial another component of this massive experiment included a large group of women who took oestrogen alone in the form of Premarin and after seven years of follow-up the women in this arm had a marginally lower incidence of breast cancer compared with the placebo group. In the American Journal of

Obstetrics and Gynaecology, April 2004, an extensive review of all the clinical trials utilising different forms of hormone replacement revealed that when oestrogen was used on its own the risk was minimal.

As it turns out the likelihood of developing breast cancer increases with age when there is not that much oestrogen floating around in the bloodstream. How can this happen when oestrogen is thought to be the prime initiator and promoter of breast cancer and increased oestrogen levels are thought to be the driving force? There are two major reasons for this. It's what happens to oestrogen that counts and it's also your body's ability to make oestrogen that can make a difference.

Your body has to deal with or eliminate oestrogen and it does this by making metabolites called 2, 4 and 16 hydroxyoestradiols. The 2 series are thought to be weak oestrogens and have the potential to be protective whereas the 4 and 16 hydroxyoestradiols are thought to be more stimulating and cancer promoting. (3) When exposed to increased free radical stresses the 4 hydroxyoestradiols form further metabolites known as the 3, 4 quinone oestrogens and it is these hormones that are really lethal to DNA leading to the type of mutations that can result in the development of cancer. (4) (5) (6) There are also enzymes, which render the 4 hydroxyoestradiols relatively harmless and these go by the name of catechol-O-methyltransferase and glutathione transferase respectively. Catechol-O-methyltransferase depends on the presence of vitamin B12 and folic acid for its activity whereas glutathione transferase relies on sufficient amounts of the antioxidant glutathione. Vitamin B12 is synthesized in your gut and is found in eggs, sardines and meat while green vegetables are good sources of folic acid. Vitamin C, N-acetylcysteine and alpha-lipoic acid are powerful antioxidants, which boost glutathione production.

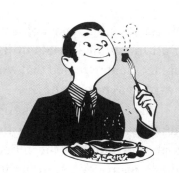

Broccoli is a cancer fighter

2 hydroxyoestradiol, the relatively harmless oestrogen metabolite, increases with regular exercise, soy, the nutrient indole-3 carbinol found in broccoli and other brassica vegetables such as cauliflower and Brussels sprouts, which is why your mother told you to eat those green vegetables, a good old cup of coffee, (1-2 cups per day will suffice) 17beta-oestradiol found in the oestrogen form of hormone replacement and a high protein diet. (7) This indicates that HRT, which includes oestrogen, can actually be protective.

The other part of this story concerns the body's ability to make oestrogen. There are two major enzymes responsible for manufacturing oestrogen one is called sulfatase and the other aromatase. This is the same aromatase that leads to the formation of oestrogen in the male body. What you need to do is limit the activity of sulfatase and aromatase. Once these enzymes are allowed endless freedom to do their thing then your body will produce too much oestrogen and you will be in trouble. It's not so much the oestrogen that is travelling around your bloodstream that does you any harm. Rather it is the oestrogen that is produced in your breast tissue as a result of the unrestrained activity of sulfatase and aromatase that can set you up to develop breast cancer. As it turns out sulfatase has the greater impact on the formation of oestrogen and here's the thing.

Research indicates that the activity of sulfatase can be brought to a halt by the action of none other than oestrogen itself. (8)This might be the very reason for the lower incidence of breast cancer in those women taking oestrogen on its own in the Women's Health Initiative Trial. (9) There is also evidence that oestrogen encourages cancer cells to commit suicide. (10) This suggests that if you are taking oestrogen this hormone might be beneficial as long as your levels remain within the healthy range. Putting the brakes on aromatase can be achieved with the help of natural substances like red grape extract otherwise known as resveratrol, flaxseeds, which you can obtain from ground flaxseeds by adding two dessertspoons of a mixture known as LSA (linseed, sunflower seeds and almonds) to your cereal in the morning and the bioflavonoid quercetin. This is very exciting news. In short HRT that includes oestrogen can be beneficial and you simply have to ensure that you are protected by all the nutrients, which support the correct disposal of this hormone.

THE OTHER HORMONES

As is the case for oestrogen excessive amounts of testosterone, DHEA and IGF-1, growth hormone's partner increase the risk for developing breast cancer. (11)(12)(13)(14) Testosterone and DHEA are precursors for oestrogen synthesis and elevated levels of these hormones provide a ready source for a hormone that you don't want too much of. IGF-1 and growth hormone on the other hand encourage cells to grow including cancer cells and there is evidence that oestrogen and IGF-1 combine quite nicely to stimulate the proliferation of tumour cells. Therefore it would make a whole lot of sense to be very respectful of these hormones once you undertake a replacement programme. If you are taking these hormones it is imperative that you have your levels checked regularly to ensure that these remain within reasonable limits. Testosterone should lie between 2-3nmol/L, DHEA 5-10umol/L and IGF-1 20-30 nmol/L.

Natural progesterone on the other hand, which is different from the progestins used in conventional hormone replacement therapy thought to be responsible for stimulating cancer cell growth, might be protective. (15) (16)

HOMOCYSTEINE

Overly high homocysteine levels have all sorts of negative ramifications for your health. There is a hypothesis which connects elevated homocysteine levels with the development of breast cancer. (17) Usually your body has no trouble dealing with homocysteine using B12 and folic acid as well as vitamin B6 to metabolise this substance to methionine or cystathione, which are relatively harmless. There is a link between B12 and folic acid deficiency and the development of breast cancer. (18) (19). With insufficient amounts of B12 and folic acid, homocysteine starts to climb and your risk of breast cancer increases. The solution is just as tidy. If you have enough vitamin B12 and folic acid your homocysteine will be looked after and one of your risk factors will fly out the window.

VITAMIN D DEFICIENCY

Vitamin D has an amazing talent for turning cancer cells into normal cells which is one of the strategies your body can adopt to stop these cells in their tracks. A deficiency of this vitamin might make it easier for cancer cells to find a home in your body. The beauty about this vitamin is that it's so easy to obtain sufficient quantities if you live in a sunny climate. 10-20 minutes of sunlight a day will provide you with all the vitamin D you need with the simple prerequisite that your kidneys and liver have the ability to potentiate this vitamin which in the normal course of things should be a mere formality.

DIET AND WEIGHT GAIN

Of all the studies that have examined the connection between dietary factors and the advancement of breast cancer well-cooked red meat is the most consistent offender. (20) This is thought to be associated with the presence of toxins known as heterocylic amines, which are damaging to your DNA. (21) Dairy especially full-cream milk also gets a bad rap in some studies although there are others especially those homing in on the benefits of low-fat milk, which indicate that this substance might in fact be protective. (23) (24) While the hormones and growth factors in dairy products might be harmful other substances found in dairy like vitamin D, calcium and conjugated linoleic acid might be beneficial. (25) (26) (27).

We used to think that all foods rich in saturated fats promote breast cancer but now research intimates that once this fat makes you put on weight problems start to mount. If you then add a diet rich in refined carbohydrates such as pastries, chocolate bars, biscuits and ice-cream, which might lead to further weight gain, you are placing yourself in danger. (28) It is the fat, which accumulates around your mid-riff that poses the most significant threat. More fat cells lead to increased production of oestrogen and the same fat cells increase your risk for developing insulin resistance. (29) Insulin is thought to stimulate cancer cells, which also thrive on the extra sugar travelling around your bloodstream. (30) Fat cells harbour those nasty inflammatory cells. The more fat you have the greater will be your body's production of inflammatory molecules which further increases your risk of developing cancer. This is why it's so important to maintain your optimal weight once you pass through menopause when weight gain can become a real issue.

ASSORTED TOXINS
ALCOHOL

For many the daily consumption of alcohol is a ritual, which has its benefits. It's relaxing and it forms the basis for communication between friends and loved ones. Then there's the antioxidants found predominantly in red wine and other alcoholic beverages that are beneficial. Unfortunately alcohol can also be a poison and for some the mere consumption of one glass per day can be enough to increase the risk of developing breast cancer.

Fortunately for most women the daily two-glass rule applies and once you exceed this the adverse effects of this substance will start to take hold especially as far as your liver, which is the main processing organ for oestrogen, is concerned. My advice is to limit your consumption of alcohol, stick to good red wine and if you can find another daily ritual, which is equally relaxing and social, so much the better.

PESTICIDES

Reports on the effects of pesticides are mixed. Some studies show that exposure to certain pesticides are toxic and increase the incidence of breast cancer while others don't. (31) (32) It would indeed be a wonderful world if everyone went out and cultivated their own little patch of garden with lots of home-grown organic fruits and vegetables free of all the additives that are applied to sustain crops and make them grow, but that's not about to happen in my lifetime. If you can locate fresh organic produce which would contain all the nourishing vitamins, minerals and antioxidants then you are doing yourself a real service. If you can't, then supplementary nutrients, which I would still recommend to everyone, are an absolute must.

HEAVY METALS

Our contact with metals such as lead, tin, mercury, cobalt, nickel, aluminium and others is constant through the food we eat, the water we drink, our daily occupations and even the air we breathe. And now studies show that these metals have the ability to make breast cancer cells multiply. (33) One of the ways to discover whether your body is affected by excessive amounts of these potential toxins is to have a hair mineral analysis, which reflects the accumulation of these substances in your cells.

Minerals such as zinc and selenium minimise the damaging effects of these metals. Even iron, which is a substance your body can't do without, has the power to inflict harm once it builds up in your system. One of the plusses of having that annoying monthly cycle is the elimination of iron when you have your period, which is probably one of the reasons for women living longer than men. Zinc and selenium also antagonise iron excess while green tea and the herb st mary's thistle can be used to improve the disposal of this metal.

ELECTROMAGNETIC RADIATION

If you live near a high-voltage power line and you have other risk factors you might want to consider relocating as there is a connection between this type of exposure and breast cancer. Equally if your occupation involves constant exposure to electromagnetic radiation, which would be the experience of switchboard operators and radiographers, then you need to pay extra special attention to the section coming up dealing with cancer prevention, which will list the steps you can take to reduce your risk. The good news about routine household exposure to this type of radiation is that reports show risks are negligible.

ANTIBIOTICS

Yes, even this seemingly harmless medication is associated with breast cancer when employed for an extended period. Recently a study in the Journal of the American Medical Association revealed that those women who took antibiotics to treat various infections had an increased risk of developing breast cancer and this risk was magnified with longer periods of antibiotic usage.

Although the reasons for this remain speculative, this phenomenon could be related to the eradication of beneficial bacteria in the bowel, which assist with the metabolism of oestrogen. This indicates that antibiotics should be used judiciously and not for lengthy periods if this can be avoided. If you are taking these medicines supplementing with probiotics such as acidophilus and bifidus will replace the good germs in your bowel that you might be losing. This will help to preserve those essential metabolic functions that might go astray.

INFLAMMATION

Inflammation is a co-conspirator in this tale with studies linking pro-inflammatory cells called cytokines with increased activity of the enzyme aromatase which in turn leads to a greater production of oestrogen. (35) (36) This sets in motion the series of events which ignite cancer cells. We don't always know what causes inflammation but there are blood tests such as the HS-CRP (highly sensitive C-reactive protein) and newer tests which measure pro-inflammatory cytokines including interleukin-6, interleukin-8 and interleukin-10 that give you some idea of the presence of inflammation in your body. Once you know it's there you can start to take the necessary steps to extinguish the smoldering flames before these intensify into a raging inferno. You'll find more about inflammation and what you can do to deal with its presence in the prevention section.

FREE RADICAL STRESS

We all get exposed to free radicals. They're unavoidable. What you can do is limit your exposure to these. Sources of these include:

- Deep fried foods
- Pesticides, herbicides and preservatives in foods
- Packaged biscuits, cakes and pastries
- Processed foods
- Exhaust fumes and other forms of industrial pollutants
- Excessive exposure to UV radiation
- Direct or passive cigarette smoke

Antioxidants found in fruit and vegetables and supplementary nutrients are your protection against the harmful effects of free radicals.

GENES

I have placed this category last only because its importance still occupies a support role when compared with the other risk factors. However with the deciphering of the genome and the ongoing research into genetic polymorphisms, which are mutations that can lead to greater exposure to oestrogen and the more dangerous metabolites such as the 3,4 quinone oestrogens, this area is going to acquire added significance.

It is also important to note that a positive genetic history and the presence of genes such as the BRCA1 and BRCA2 mutations merely increase your risk but they are not an absolute guarantee that you will get cancer. If you do have first degree relatives with breast cancer, especially if they developed this disease before the age of 50, then you really should have more aggressive screening measures including blood tests for the above mentioned genetic mutations, regular physical examination plus mammographic screening and you need to pay special attention to the other risk factors and the means at your disposal for preventing breast cancer which encompasses the next section.

No single risk factor is a surefire certainty that you will get breast cancer. It is probably the combination of the excesses of each of these that conspires to disrupt DNA replication in such a way that cancer cells are born which go on to replicate and multiply. This process takes many years to come to fruition, which suggests that you can intervene aggressively to derail this mechanism before it establishes itself in your body. It goes without saying that the most effective course of action would be to limit any risk factor so that it does you no harm.

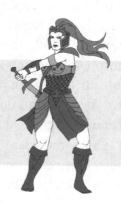

Defend Yourself
against Breast Cancer

RISK FACTORS FOR BREAST CANCER

- Over-exposure to oestrogen
- The metabolites of oestrogen including 4 and 16 hydroxyoestradiols and the 3,4 quinone oestrogens
- Overactivity of aromatase, the enzyme which produces oestrogen
- Progestins employed in hormone replacement therapy
- Free radical stress
- High testosterone, DHEA and IGF-1 levels
- Deficiencies of vitamin B12, folic acid and vitamin D
- Elevated homocysteine levels
- Well-cooked red meat
- Full-cream milk
- Obesity with increased ingestion of animal fats and high-glycaemic index foods
- Insulin resistance
- The consumption of more than two alcoholic drinks per day
- Pesticides
- Heavy metals including lead, tin, mercury, cobalt, nickel and aluminium
- Electromagnetic radiation
- Prolonged use of antibiotics
- Inflammation
- Mutations of the BRCA-1 and BRCA-2 genes

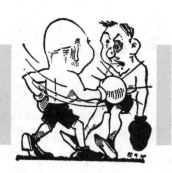

Melatonin is an
antioxidant
heavy weight

PREVENTING BREAST CANCER

HORMONES

Melatonin, thyroid hormones, progesterone, DHEA and oestriol (the weaker oestrogen) offer the most promise of preventing breast cancer. Of all of these melatonin probably fares the best. This hormone is an antioxidant heavyweight and an impressive stimulator of the immune system. Melatonin is produced in darkness and studies show that the blind and those who live in Nordic countries where winter darkness is protracted have a lower incidence of breast cancer. (37) Conversely shift workers who are exposed to nighttime light suffer from an increased risk of developing breast cancer. My advice is to have your melatonin levels measured via a salivary assay performed just before you go to sleep at night and if this is low boosting this hormone might provide you with some protection.

Thyroid hormones are also worth a look in with evidence that T3 the dominant thyroid hormone has the ability to inhibit cancer cells indicating that having your thyroid hormones measured and optimising your levels of these would be advisable. (38) Progesterone is the late Dr John Lee's golden hormone with the ability to prevent cancer in a host of ways by limiting the negative effects of excess cortisol, the stress hormone, augmenting thyroid hormone, stimulating the immune system and halting the growth of cancer cells. (39)

While some studies do support Dr Lee's claims others seem to indicate that progesterone might not exactly be the wonder hormone that it's made out to be with some even showing that this hormone encourages cancer cells to multiply suggesting that you need to maintain your progesterone levels within healthy limits rather than risk overexposure to this hormone. (40)(41)(42).

DHEA's contribution is equally complex. Animal research points to the protective effects of this hormone. However postmenopausal women who experience heightened exposure to DHEA are at increased risk if they have low oestrogen levels. With the documented beneficial effects that this hormone brings to bear on the immune system it might be worthwhile augmenting your levels if they are low. However, it is also important to ensure that your other hormones are in balance when you enhance this hormone as elevated DHEA and low oestrogen levels can lead to difficulties. Even oestriol, which is thought to have an impeccable pedigree with regard to preventing breast cancer, has been shown in one study to slightly increase the risk. (43) The bottom line is if you are taking hormones make sure that your levels remain within healthy limits otherwise you could get yourself into trouble

THE VITAMINS

Folic acid and vitamin D are the standout performers as far as breast cancer prevention is concerned. Those women who like their alcohol need to pay special attention as your risk increases if you consume more than 15g of alcohol per day, which would be the equivalent of the two-glass limit. (44) This is because alcohol opposes the action of folic acid, which amplifies your need for this nutrient. 3-5 mg per day is a reasonable dose of folic acid. Vitamin D can be obtained from sunlight as well as tuna, cod, egg yolk, fortified orange juice and sprouted seeds. (45) Carotenoids, which are found in carrots, pumpkins, apricots and leafy green vegetables also have a role to play especially when combined with docosahexanoic acid found in fish. (46)

Unfortunately Vitamins C and E don't fare so well with not much support for their beneficiary powers from scientific studies, although there is some cheer for cancer sufferers with evidence that these nutrients do reduce cancer recurrence.

DIET AND EXERCISE

Here the advice is delightfully simple. Eat lots of fruit and vegetables. If you can, locate organic produce or grow your own. Maintain your optimal weight and resist those fat-laden and sugar-filled items that fast-food outlets are so adept at including in their daily fare. And then you have to exercise. You need to put aside 3-4 hours per week and you have to exercise at moderate to vigorous levels, which means generating a sweat. If you're not sweating it probably means that you're not expending enough effort.

THE SPECIAL NUTRIENTS

SOY

Soy has the potential to prevent breast cancer. However, and this is vitally important, there are major stipulations. You have to consume soy products early on in life to obtain any protective advantage and you have to ingest predominantly fermented soy in the form of miso and tempeh to gain the real benefits. This is probably why Asian populations enjoy the protective effects that soy has to offer. In these cultures the children are consumers and they eat the health-giving form of this substance. It's no use wolfing down sizeable amounts of soy in your forties and fifties because this is when this substance can actually do you some harm.

If there isn't much oestrogen in your body soy can actually increase your levels of this hormone and in some cases this can provide fertile ground for cancer growth. Soy can stimulate cancer cells and this can be a real disaster for cancer sufferers. Tamoxifen is also inhibited by the presence of soy. My advice is to stick with miso, tempeh and tofu, have 2-3 serves per week and the earlier you start enjoying this nutrient the better.

FLAXSEED

Although there is no documented evidence that this substance actually prevents breast cancer it does limit oestrogen levels in the breast due to its powerful inhibitory effects on aromatase. Aromatase inhibitors are now becoming one of the primary means for actually treating breast cancer and in flaxseed you have a natural substance, which functions like the medications used to achieve this outcome without any nasty side-effects. This nutrient therefore has the potential for both prevention and treatment. Adding two dessertspoons of ground flaxseed to your breakfast cereal on a daily basis will furnish you with all the protection you need.

FISH OILS

Until now eating 2-3 serves of fish per week has widely been viewed as a wise investment in your health with regard to preventing cancer and heart disease. A recent study out of Denmark has shed some rather disturbing light on this notion with the news that rather than being protective higher intakes of fish are actually associated with a greater incidence of breast cancer. (47) Just when you thought that you could at least count on fish to bring home the bacon along comes a study to prove you're wrong. If you can't eat well-cooked red meat, full-cream milk is not a good idea, you have to stay away from saturated fat and sweet foods, soy has its downside, alcohol could be dangerous and now even fish, the last refuge of the health-conscious is off limits then what is left for you?

Being a devout vegetarian I'm obviously tempted to say there's still good old fruit and vegetables that are full of those lifesaving antioxidants. To give fish its due the negative outcome in this study might have had a lot to do with the contaminants polluting the waters around Denmark although the authors appeared to discount this. I still believe that if you consume the smaller fish such as sardines and flounder then you shouldn't have to deal with harmful substances such as mercury and the assorted pesticides accumulating in the larger fish.

It might be better to go directly for eicosapentanoic acid (EPA) and docosahexanoic acid (DHA), the healthy oils found in fish, as these are the ingredients that contain all the anti-inflammatory properties. If the manufacturer is reliable, EPA and DHA in supplementary form are usually free of any contaminating substances. One gram per day of EPA and DHA would be a healthy dose.

ANTI-INFLAMMATORY AGENTS

Aspirin and non-steroidal anti-inflammatory drugs (NSAIDs) are widely used to treat arthritis pain and in the case of aspirin to thin the blood. Recently and quite fortuitously it was discovered that women who take these medications for long periods of time have a lower incidence of breast cancer. As inflammation is thought to be one of the principal instigators of the cancer process short-circuiting this train of events might have a lot to do with the serendipitous benefits of these medications. Unfortunately NSAIDs and aspirin have the ability to erode the lining of your bowel, which could cause bleeding and ulcers. Going to your local pharmacy and loading up on these drugs might not be the most prudent course of action.

Long before the pharmaceutical companies came along nature in its wisdom had formulated a whole range of natural anti-inflammatory substances, which operate in a similar fashion to NSAIDs and aspirin without the damaging side-effects. Ginger, turmeric, rosemary, oregano, green tea, resveratrol (red grape extract) and the omega-3 fatty acid DHA all have the power to halt inflammation in its tracks and including these in your diet might be a substantial investment in your health.

GREEN TEA

I'm a great endorser of green tea. Aside from having anti-inflammatory properties this substance is a powerful anti-cancer agent. There's an old adage, which goes along the lines of: if something tastes really nice it's probably not that good for you whereas an unpleasant taste usually indicates it's very healthy. This might not always be true but in the case of green tea I regularly have to endure complaints about the taste of this beverage. I have an inventive if not quirky way round this. To dilute the unpleasant taste of green tea, try using either dandelion coffee and/or rooibos tea (also known as red bush) as a chaser. These have a delightful taste and dandelion is good for your liver while rooibos is antioxidant rich.

The other option is black tea, which is derived from the

same source as green tea but has a lower complement of antioxidants. Although the advantages are not as clear-cut as they are for green tea one study has shown that Asian-American women who have a reduced propensity to metabolise black tea, in other words they retain this substance for a longer period of time in their bodies, have a lower incidence of breast cancer. (48) However, if you want to go where the real money is then saddle up with green tea. The more cups you drink the greater the protection.

RESVERATROL

This is one of my favourite nutrients. There's nothing that this substance cannot do ranging from its anti-inflammatory powers to its ability to inhibit cancer cells and limit the effects of aromatase, which reduces oestrogen levels. To top it all resveratrol even contributes to longevity. This is why the French benefit so much from red wine despite their appalling eating habits. It's the skin of the red grapes, which are resveratrol's source. Because of the limitations of alcohol supplementary resveratrol would be a more favourable choice and a dose of 5mg daily would have the potential to be protective.

INDOLE-3 CARBINOL

This is the substance that is derived from brassica vegetables like broccoli, sprouts and cabbage, which makes the weaker, more beneficial 2 hydroxyoestrogens. In animals indole-3 carbinol has been shown to prevent the occurrence of breast cancer. To obtain the protective effects of this nutrient you would have to eat a truckload of brassica vegetables and if you're struggling with the taste of green tea then broccoli isn't exactly going to tantalise your taste buds. The supplement might be a better idea. Indole-3 carbinol is converted in your body to another tongue twister, which goes by the name of diindolylmethane or DIM for short and the companies that market these two substances are involved in an infernal bunfight to assert the superiority of their product. There is one study which shows that while preventing breast cancer indole-3 carbinol also has the potential to induce liver and bowel cancer. (49.) This would seem to make DIM the preferred option.

Like soy, brassica vegetables and DIM might have a more profound influence when used at an earlier age and there is a study indicating that genistein found in soy and DIM work synergistically to encourage cancer cells to commit suicide. (50) 300mg daily of DIM would be an effective dose.

IODINE AND SELENIUM

These are minerals, which are critically important for the function of the thyroid gland. This is the gland, which revs up your immune system to protect you against breast cancer. It is not uncommon to be deficient in these minerals and if you find that your thyroid blood test is in the normal to low zone and your morning temperature is sub-optimal then taking kelp, which is a good source of iodine, might help to boost your thyroid function.

Equally selenium, which is found in Brazil nuts, cabbage, garlic, onions and seafood, might need to be supplemented to guarantee that you have adequate supplies of this mineral. 200micrograms daily would be a reliable dose.

MAMMOGRAPHY and THERMOGRAPHY

There is a raging debate regarding the value of utilising mammography as a screening device for the early detection of beast cancer. One school of thought endorses this approach claiming that it picks up tumours before the disease entrenches itself in the body leading to the kind of treatment which affords a better prognosis. The alternate point of view argues that mammography is no better than a regular self-examination for detecting breast cancer and that this type of technology doesn't improve survival rates for those with a positive diagnosis. Added to which there is the problem of regular exposure to radiation and the discomfort of this examination.

In defence of mammography there are many experts who are at pains to inform us that there has been a substantial reduction in cancer mortality as a result of screening with this technology and that women over the age of 40 should consider having this investigation every two years. (51) (52) Australian experts claim that there is insufficient evidence to support screening between the ages of 40-49 and have suggested that this should be commenced from the age of 50. Ultrasound can be used as an adjunct to mammography, and while this detects additional cancers, there is also the problem of additional false positives. Magnetic resonance imaging (MRI) has recently been introduced which might have better sensitivity than mammography but lower specificity. This has yet to be embraced in the wider medical arena.

Other technologies have also been gaining momentum in the race to discover the best method for identifying breast cancer. One of these is thermography. This measures differences in heat emission from normal tissue and breast cancers. The area in which this investigation is done is cooled with fans that lower room temperature. This has the effect of reducing the blood supply to normal tissue because vessels constrict when exposed to cold temperatures while tumors remain hot and can be detected by infrared scanners. There are claims by physicians who incorporate this technology that thermography is highly sensitive and can identify 95% of breast cancers with 90% accuracy. (53) To say the least this statistic is highly impressive. Because younger women have dense breast tissue, detection of tumours by means of mammography can be difficult. However this is not a problem with thermographic screening which also involves no radiation exposure or breast compression. Women can begin having thermograms from the age of 25, which might allow for detection of suspicious areas long before mammography isolates a tumour. Thermography has yet to become a mainstream investigation and I have to say that I still consider routine mammograms combined with regular self-examination to be the best current option. However if you have a positive family history then commencing periodic thermography at a much younger age than that for mammography might indeed be beneficial.

Here is a list of the major players, which might help to prevent breast cancer

- Melatonin
- Thyroid hormones
- Progesterone
- DHEA
- Oestriol
- Fruit and Vegetables
- Folic Acid
- Vitamin D
- Carotenoids
- Soy

- EPA
- DHA
- Flaxseed
- Green tea
- Resveratrol
- DIM
- Iodine
- Selenium

TREATING BREAST CANCER

Linda was 39 when she began to notice the small lump in her breast, which she thought felt a little different. After ignoring it for a while she decided that it was about time she told her doctor just so that he could reassure her there was nothing wrong. When the biopsy returned a positive diagnosis she didn't quite hear the doctor telling her that she had breast cancer. Two weeks later she'd had the operation, which saw to it that the tumour had been removed, but then it turned out her lymph nodes were infiltrated with the cancer. I saw Linda after she'd had radiotherapy and was commencing her first course of chemotherapy.

When I was a medical student attending ward rounds I don't ever remember the doctors referring to cancer by its actual name. We used the words 'growth', 'carcinoma' and occasionally even the quaint phrase 'something there' as if using a euphemism would make the real thing go away.

Receiving a cancer diagnosis has to be just about the worst news anyone can get. Far and away it has to be the biggest health challenge of them all. Fortunately Linda wasn't about to accept that conventional medical treatments were the only options available to her. By the time I got to see her she had recovered enough from the shock to be inquisitive about all the other therapies that she could utilise in addition to the medical treatments she was receiving

Here's what's on offer.

THE HORMONES

Melatonin is the hormone with the most potential. This is the hormone that is an antioxidant powerhouse with a mountain of immune-boosting capacity. Aside from one study, which reveals that melatonin isn't beneficial, there are a number of animal trials and cell culture studies indicating that this hormone is highly effective against breast cancer as well as assisting tamoxifen. (53) (54) (55) (56) One of the problems with chemotherapy is the awful side effects and melatonin has the ability to reduce these and improves the survival chances of those who have added this hormone to their regimen. (57) There is also evidence that melatonin combines effectively with vitamin D3, linoleic acid found in fish and flaxseed oil, and retinoic acid, the vitamin A derivative, to inhibit the growth of cancer cells. (58) (59) As melatonin can also be used to treat insomnia, a good initial dose would be 3mg taken just before sleeping and this can be increased to as much as 20mg.

Although there are some animal and cell culture studies which show that DHEA and testosterone are effective inhibitors of breast cancer cells, these treatments have yet to be widely embraced by mainstream medicine. (60) This is probably because of the fear that these hormones have the capacity to increase oestrogen levels, which could make matters worse. I must confess to sharing this apprehension and therefore I too am very reluctant to incorporate these hormones as a therapeutic strategy.

VITAMINS AND ANTIOXIDANTS

One of the enduring controversies about vitamins and antioxidants is whether they actually make a difference and this is especially true with regard to cancer therapy. This issue is even more critical when you consider that there are a number of experts out there who insist that these substances interfere with cancer treatments such as chemotherapy and radiation therapy. As long as you have a healthy diet and eat everything in moderation, they say, it's pretty much all you need. To this you can add a multivitamin if you have to, but large doses of vitamins are an absolute no-no because not only may they harm normal cells but they may also help cancer cells become resistant to conventional treatments. The issue here is that chemotherapy and radiation therapy rely on the generation of free radicals to kill cancer cells and antioxidants that neutralise free radicals would undermine this process. This is one point of view and it's the position that most oncologists appear to be taking. Indeed the recommendation of the American Institute for Cancer Research is to caution patients against the use of megadoses of vitamin and mineral supplements as the evidence that confirms their safety and benefits is limited. (61)

The other perspective asserts that for the most part chemotherapy and radiation therapy operate by damaging the DNA of cancer cells rather than through the promulgation of free radicals. (62) In order to increase the vulnerability of cancer cells to the above treatments they need to be dividing rapidly and the more free radicals you have the slower cancer cells actually replicate. In other words, by reducing free radical stress antioxidants assist chemotherapy and radiation therapy rather than rendering them less effective.

American expert Kedar Prasad from the University of Colorado who has researched extensively on the pros and cons of antioxidant use during cancer treatments supports this perspective and he suggests that large doses of certain vitamins and minerals should be taken prior to, during and after these treatments to optimise their efficacy while reducing all the debilitating side-effects that accompany standard therapy.

The only antioxidants that you should omit during radiotherapy and chemotherapy are N-acetylcysteine, selenium and alpha-lipoic acid as these have the ability to increase the glutathione (another antioxidant) content of cancer cells making them more resistant to conventional treatments. (63) (64) Incidentally Linda decided to opt for the more conservative approach by omitting any natural remedies during her conventional radiation and chemotherapy treatments and commenced these once her regulation therapies were completed.

The point about vitamins is that they work as a team. Ten years ago a group of scientists in Denmark followed the progress of 32 patients who had breast cancer, which had spread to their lymph nodes. They received routine surgical and therapeutic treatments and they then went on to take a combination of nutritional antioxidants including vitamins C and E, betacarotene, omega 6 and omega 3-fatty acids, selenium and coenzyme Q10 as well as a B vitamin and a mineral complex. At the end of the 18 months none of the patients had died, none showed any signs of distant metastases or spread of their cancer, their quality of life had improved and six had gone into partial remission. Although 18 months is not an extensive period of time this is a pretty impressive return on a rather simple antioxidant programme.

Sadly, a longer trial, which investigated the effects of an assortment of vitamins including beta-carotene, vitamin C, niacin, selenium, coenzyme Q10, and zinc on survival and recurrence in breast cancer sufferers revealed that the treatment group fared no better than those who did not take these supplements. To sway the pendulum back in favour of vitamin supplementation a 12 year follow-up to ascertain those factors related to breast cancer survival showed that those women who took vitamin C and vitamin E supplements for more than three years had a lower recurrence rate of their cancer and reduced disease-related mortality. (65)(66)

If you look at all the scientific evidence you will find that there are a multitude of studies which show that vitamins and antioxidants effectively kill cancer cells at least in the test tube and as far as animal experimentation is concerned. Vitamins C, D, and E, tocotrienols (vitamin E like substances), retinoic acid (a derivative of vitamin A), lycopene, quercetin, selenium and coenzyme Q10 all feature prominently in this area. (67) (68) (69) (70)(71) (72) (73)(74)

Vitamins might help to conquer cancer

I'm going to side with the positive side of this story and endorse these substances as legitimate contenders in the ongoing war against cancer. It would be nice if we had substantial scientific evidence for this but for the time being all I can say is that there is some justification for this approach and more would be comforting. To get the maximum effect you have to take combinations of vitamins and antioxidants. They don't work that well if you use them individually. Shortly I'll provide you with a list of all these remedies plus their dosages, which you can incorporate in your treatment regimen.

HERBAL MEDICINES AND OTHER REMEDIES

The advantage of most of these substances is that their principal function is to fortify the immune system, which allows the body to deal more effectively with cancer cells. Ultimately this should make it far easier for chemotherapy to do its thing while at the same time reducing any damage to normal cells.

You've already met resveratrol. This is the nutrient that has all the smarts as far as inhibiting breast cancer cells is concerned. A good dose of resveratrol would be 20mg daily. Aside from preventing breast cancer green tea cuts off the blood supply to cancer cells, prevents them from spreading and encourages them to commit suicide - not a bad recipe for terminating cancer cells. If you can get to enjoy the taste, 4-6 cups per day would provide you with a healthy dose of green tea. Alternatively green tea can be obtained in capsule form. A therapeutic daily dose would be 500-1000mg.

Calcium-D-glucarate is the salt of D-glucaric acid, a substance that is found in oranges, apples, grapefruit and cruciferous vegetables. Together with retinoic acid this nutrient inhibits tumour growth in rats and humans. It also makes cancer cells change into normal cells, helps the liver to get rid of toxins and inhibits an enzyme called beta-glucuronidase which lowers oestrogen levels. The recommended daily dosage of calcium-D-glucarate is 1500-3000mg.

Maitake MD-fraction is a medicinal mushroom that operates primarily by boosting the immune system and increasing natural killer and cytotoxic T-cells which allows for more efficient elimination of cancer cells. In a Japanese trial 11 out of 16 breast cancer sufferers experienced significant improvements when they received this compound with some even going into regression. (76) One 41 year - old patient who was being treated with tamoxifen and 5 fluorouracil developed metastases but when she took 125mg MD-fraction together with 4 grams of the whole maitake extract her tumour miraculously disappeared. Hair loss, nausea and the decline in white blood cells, the traditional stumbling blocks of chemotherapy can be significantly reduced with this substance. Commercial preparations of the MD-fraction typically contain 3-25mg of the standardised extract.

Astragalus is another one of my favourite herbal remedies. This herb has been used for centuries by the Chinese and its strength lies in its ability to boost the immune system and to potentiate the activity of chemotherapeutic agents while at the same time reducing the toxicities of these medicines. 8-10grms per day would constitute a good therapeutic dose.

Tahitian noni juice, used by the Polynesians for over 2000 years, is another herb with impeccable immune enhancing credentials. Enhancing the effectiveness of chemotherapy, inhibiting cancer cells when they begin to multiply and switching off those inflammatory cells which help tumours to entrench themselves are just some of the ways that this herb can help you to defeat cancer. You need to take large amounts of noni to achieve an effective dose. 1 litre of the liquid or ten 1200mg capsules taken in divided doses daily would provide you with a reasonable initial dose, which can then be reduced over time.

Curcumin is the herb that gives curry its piquant edge. Its ability to invigorate your taste buds is matched by its potential to inhibit the proliferation of cancer cells and cut off their blood supply once they start to spread their wings. Curcumin is a herb with lots of promise for fighting cancer but there is one small proviso with taking this substance. There is one study which suggests that curcumin can interfere with chemotherapeutic medications like cyclophophamide and therefore it might be a good idea to delay utilising this remedy until you have completed your chemotherapy treatment. The recommended dosage for curcumin in capsule form is 200-400mg taken one to three times daily.

For cancer cells to grow and spread they need a blood supply and what they do is express tiny protein molecules on their surface, which are like calling cards that invite the blood vessels to supply them with nutrients. Modified citrus pectin, which is derived from the pulp of citrus fruits, has the ingenious capability of latching on to these surface proteins and disrupting their activity so that they are no longer able to attract a blood supply. This effectively prevents cancer cells from metastasising. In test tube conditions modified citrus pectin has been shown to prevent breast cancer cells from attaching to the walls of blood vessels, which stopped these cells from disseminating. The recommended dose is 15-20grms daily

THE DIET

Cancer cells thrive on sugar and they live in an anaerobic environment. Anaerobic means without oxygen and this is the type of biochemical pathway your body chooses if your cells aren't functioning smoothly and don't have all the nutrients they need to utilise oxygen efficiently to provide you with energy. There are all sorts of cancer friendly diets out there but I suggest that you keep it simple and apply the same dietary principles that have been alluded to throughout this book. This should see to it that your cells are operating to their maximal capacity.

Consume a healthy amount of fruits and vegetables and if you can, eat fresh organic produce that's in season and keep some of it raw which helps to preserve your enzymes. Enzymes don't only assist with digestion but they also help you to fight cancer by enhancing your immune system, encouraging cancer cells to differentiate or change into normal cells and they prevent these cells from spreading.

Obtain your protein from eggs, nuts, seeds, small fish and some meat if you have to. I have a leaning towards vegetarianism but this is not absolutely essential. Whey powder is a complete source of protein and this substance also has the advantage of depleting cancer cells of glutathione, which makes them more vulnerable to chemotherapy. Stay with low-glycaemic index carbohydrates, resist all those sugary treats, avoid any foods to which you are allergic, cut back on animal fats especially dairy products and maintain your ideal weight. Supplementing your diet with B vitamins, magnesium and zinc will help to provide those nutrients that preserve healthy aerobic metabolism. Cut out alcohol, at least for the time being, and exercise 4-5 times per week if you can.

Ensure that you are well hydrated and introduce juicing into your daily regimen. I'm a great fan of wheatgrass juice, which tastes a tad worse than green tea but also has a host of nutritious properties and you can always chase it down with a cocktail of apple, carrot, celery and ginger juice. Beetroot juice is another must for the taste aficionados.

Aside from green tea there is also essiac tea, a combination of four herbs including burdock, Indian rhubarb, sorrel and slippery elm embraced by a Canadian nurse in 1922 when one of her patients claimed that this formula given to her by a traditional native American healer cured her breast cancer. While there is considerable anecdotal evidence that this tea has made a difference to countless cancer sufferers and that burdock and Indian rhubarb do have anti-cancer effects there aren't really any clinical trials backing up these reports. This doesn't mean that this tea won't do you any good. It merely indicates that the science behind this formulation isn't as rock solid as we'd like it to be and this can be a problem that crops up with natural remedies from time to time.

Here then is a summary of all the hormones and nutrients that will help you to take a stand against your cancer. These remedies are not meant to replace conventional therapy rather they are intended to reinforce medical treatments while reducing what can sometimes be crippling side effects.

Natural remedies for treating breast cancer

- Melatonin 3-20mg taken at night
- Vitamin C 6-10grms daily
- Vitamin D3 2000-4000i.u. daily
- Retinoic acid 20-40mg daily
- Vitamin E succinate 400mg daily
- Vitamin E tocotrienols 50mg daily
- Lycopene 10-20mg daily
- Quercetin 1000-1500mg daily
- Selenium 200microgrms daily
- Coenzyme Q10 100mg three times daily
- Resveratrol 20mg daily
- Green tea capsules 500-1000mg daily
- Calcium-D-glucarate 1500-3000mg daily
- Maitake MD-fraction 3-25mg daily
- Astragalus 8-10 grams daily
- Tahitian noni juice 100-500mls daily
- Curcumin capsules 200-400mg one three times daily
- Modified citrus pectin 15-20grms daily

You might think you'll become a walking dispensary if you take all these remedies but if you want to defeat cancer you do need a formidable team of supplements. Aside from a few omissions this is the regimen that Linda is on at the time of writing this segment and although it is early days so far she is doing very well.

As indicated earlier she elected not to take any of the above during her chemotherapy treatment and we also decided to omit selenium from the early stages of her programme as this nutrient can increase the glutathione content of cancer cells which might make them more resilient.

PROSTATE CANCER

There are some remarkable similarities between breast and prostate cancer. The incidence of both is approximately one in ten. The likelihood of developing these diseases increases with ageing and they share many common risk factors. Where they do part company is with respect to how these cancers are treated. It is said that most men die with their prostate cancer rather than because of their cancer. In other words this cancer usually develops in the latter part of a man's life and grows so slowly that other diseases are likely to be more lethal than this relatively innocuous malady. Studies show that nine out of ten men diagnosed with early prostate cancer can expect to live for at least ten years without succumbing to this disease. There is also good evidence to show that for this early form of prostate cancer the policy of 'watchful waiting' or no medical treatment leads to the same life expectancy as that for surgery or radiotherapy for at least the first five years after the diagnosis has been made.

This begs the question as to whether it's worthwhile even knowing that you have prostate cancer and whether you should have regular blood tests which raise the alarm bells that something untoward is happening. The truth is that in the minority of cases some prostate cancers can be aggressive and they can spread rather rapidly. When this happens effective treatment becomes extremely difficult. The problem is it is not always possible to predict, with 100% certainty, which cancers have the potential to be harmful and which will meander along without doing much damage.

Try telling that to David who was in his early fifties and going along quite nicely without any major health problems except for some concerns about his weight problem and a rather poor diet when his doctor advised him that this might be a good time to have a blood test which measured his PSA (prostate-specific antigen). His doctor explained that this was round about the time when it became prudent to have annual blood tests which evaluated the PSA, a form of screening test for prostate cancer and that any abnormalities in this evaluation would suggest that all was not well with his prostate. This sounded like a reasonable test to have.

Naturally David wasn't expecting any bad news and so he hardly heard his doctor informing him that his blood test result was suspiciously high and that he should consult with a specialist as soon as possible. Two weeks later and with a comparable blood test result the specialist recommended that David have a biopsy of his prostate, which did indeed reveal that he had prostate cancer.

It's exceedingly difficult to imagine what must have been going through David's mind when he received this information. Here he is a seemingly well, albeit overweight, 52 year-old who is suddenly staring down the barrel of an extremely serious illness. The bright light if there is one in this story was the news that the cancer cells were only present in some of the biopsy specimens and it appeared that these cells were in the early stages of development. This suggested that medical treatment would have a good chance of eradicating the cancer and that the prognosis was a good one.

When I saw David he was still coming to grips with his diagnosis and while he was probably going to proceed with surgery he wanted to know whether there were any alternative strategies that he could adopt to help beat his cancer. In this scenario David's predicament can hardly be viewed as benign. It's far safer to adopt those measures which will help you to prevent prostate cancer than to wait for that gut-wrenching moment when you receive the bad news. Here's what we've discovered to date about preventing prostate cancer including all the alternative treatment possibilities for managing this disease.

RISK FACTORS FOR PROSTATE CANCER

THE HORMONES

The incidence of prostate cancer increases dramatically with ageing. Testosterone is the major hormone which stimulates prostate growth, however, most prostate cancers occur when testosterone levels are on the decline. In the prostate testosterone makes oestrogen and another stronger male hormone called dihydrotestosterone. While testosterone could be a minor player it is thought that oestrogen is the major initiator of prostate cancer with dihydrotestosterone also having a subsidiary role. Although testosterone levels tend to go down with ageing oestrogen levels stay constant or even increase and it is oestrogen that makes the prostate more sensitive to testosterone. It is the oestrogen dominant environment with an increase in the ratio of oestrogen to testosterone and dihydrotestosterone that proves a fertile ground for the development of cancer. Testosterone and dihydrotestosterone need to be around to facilitate the process but it is oestrogen that is the primary initiator of those cellular changes that result in the march towards cancer. When rats are given either testosterone or dihydrotestosterone, cancer does not manifest that often. However, when testosterone is combined with oestrogen, prostate cancer occurs in every one of those animals. Oestrogen on its own doesn't generate cancer either and it's clear that it's the team efforts of male and female hormones that initiate cancer. In the presence of testosterone and dihydrotestosterone oestrogen activates inflammatory cells, which in turn increase free radicals and these are thought to set the cancer process in motion.

It's the same story once again, hormonal imbalance fuelling inflammation and free radical stress, which switches on cancer. Amazingly excessive exposure to testosterone and oestrogen exposure in the womb also has an impact on prostate cancer development in later life. African-American men have a higher incidence of prostate cancer than their Caucasian counterparts and this is thought to be at least partly due to the higher levels of maternal testosterone and oestrogen that they experience during this gestational phase.

What's even more fascinating is the research which reveals that it is the same oestrogen metabolites which wreak havoc on the female body that have the ability to provoke cancer in the male prostate. Oestrogen undergoes a similar metabolic process in the male body forming 2, 4 and 16 hydroxyoestrogens. The 2 metabolites are the weaker oestrogens while the 4 and 16 series are thought to be more stimulating. It is the oestrogen-3,4-quinones, the by-products of the 4 hydroxyoestrogens that are the real bad guys and they cause the same DNA damage and initiate cancer in the same way that they seem able to do in breast tissue. In the rat model it is the dual administration of testosterone with these types of oestrogens that leads to cancer.

This means that the same weapons that protect women against these harmful hormones can be used to fortify men.

By having sufficient quantities of vitamins B12, folic acid and glutathione these destructive oestrogens can be shunted down those metabolic pathways, which render them harmless. To raise your glutathione levels you need to take additional alpha-lipoic acid.

Aside from the oestrogen-3,4-quinones, the 16 hydroxyoestrogens also pose somewhat of a threat while the 2 hydroxyoestrogens are protective. It is the indole-3 carbinols found in the cruciferous vegetables such as broccoli, cabbage and cauliflower which increase 2 hydroxyoestrogens and reduce 16 hydroxyoestrogens.

If oestrogen is the major instigator of cancer cell growth and testosterone and dihydrotestosterone are promoting agents, can elevated levels of these latter two hormones also trigger the development of cancer? While studies show a connection between high dihydrotestosterone and testosterone levels and prostate cancer there is no evidence that these hormones initiate this process. (78) (79) (80) (81) (82) (83).

One year-long trial, which incorporated testosterone replacement therapy to treat men who were at high risk for the development of prostate cancer, demonstrated no increase in cancer risk. (84) In fact, there are even clinical trials which reveal that low levels of testosterone are connected with this disease and even lead to cancers with a worse prognosis. (85) This makes sense when we consider the fact that prostate cancer manifests itself at that time of life when testosterone levels are low. However, to be safe if you are on testosterone treatment make sure that you aren't getting too much testosterone and that you aren't overly stimulated by dihydrotestosterone. In a similar fashion to the action of oestrogen, excessive levels of these hormones can spark off free radical processes, which might make your cells more vulnerable to tumour development.

Both growth hormone and DHEA have to be treated with the same respect accorded to testosterone. This is because high levels of IGF-1, growth hormone's accomplice, have been linked to an increased prostate cancer risk. (86) (87) It stands to reason that growth hormone which encourages cells to develop, hence its name, might equally stimulate cancer cell growth. This is why extreme caution should be exercised if you take growth hormone when your body is still producing reasonable amounts of this hormone. While there is no evidence that growth hormone replacement actually causes prostate cancer, if you are on a course of growth hormone therapy then you need to have your IGF-1 levels constantly monitored to ensure that they remain within healthy limits which would be 20-30nmol/Litre.

DHEA supplementation demands similar vigilance. Some experts will tell you that DHEA inhibits prostate cancer development in rats and even lowers the PSA score while others will claim that this hormone is actually associated with prostate cancer. (88) (89) Either way what DHEA can do in men is make oestrogen as well as testosterone. In some men the tendency is to manufacture more oestrogen whereas in others there is a leaning towards testosterone. We already know that heightened oestrogen exposure can spell trouble and the effects of testosterone can also creep up on you if your levels are too high. If you need DHEA and you commence treatment with this hormone then you need to have your levels checked regularly along with oestrogen and testosterone. DHEA should not go much higher than 10-13nmol/L and oestrogen should remain within the 80-110nmol/L range while testosterone should not exceed 30-33nmol/L.

VITAMIN DEFICIENCIES

Vitamin D stands alone in the spotlight as the vitamin that is central to the prevention of prostate cancer. This is the vitamin that you get from sunlight as well as fish oil, egg yolks and fortified milk. Just to jog your memory this vitamin can prevent cancer in many different ways. Vitamin D can derail the cell cycle which prevents cancer cells from multiplying, encourage cancer cells to commit suicide, inhibit the expression of the enzyme that immortalises cancer cells called tolemerase, cut off the blood supply to cancer cells, switch on growth regulators such as IGF binding protein 3 (IGFBP-3) that limit cancer cell growth and change cancer cells back to normal cells. If ever there was a substance worth having around surely vitamin D would have to be the number one contender.

While we are still struggling to define the precise cause of prostate cancer it is apparent that race, age and geography are unifying risk factors. The common denominator for all of these appears to be the deficiency of vitamin D. Prostate cancer is more common in northern regions of the world such as North America and North-western Europe where sunlight and vitamin D is less accessible. The highest incidence of prostate cancer in the world is found in African American males who coincidentally have high levels of the pigment forming melanin in their skins, which reduces vitamin D synthesis. Less vitamin D is manufactured with ageing when the rates of prostate cancer escalate.

While a deficiency of vitamin D can increase your risk for developing prostate cancer, a recent Scandinavian study has demonstrated that excessive levels of vitamin D can also make you more vulnerable. (93) To obtain the protective benefits of vitamin D this substance has to go through a series of empowering biochemical processes in your body.

Paradoxically high vitamin D concentrations actually interfere with these metabolic pathways, which prevents you from getting the form of vitamin D that you really need. Avid consumption of dairy products might have the potential to suppress vitamin D production, which I'm going to discuss shortly. Maintaining your vitamin D levels within the normal range, which is 40-60nmol/L, would give you the most benefits and all you have to do to achieve these levels is enjoy 20 minutes of sunlight daily. This also means that spending long periods of time in the sun might also lead to excessive vitamin D levels, which is equally not beneficial.

DIET AND WEIGHT GAIN

If you consume an excessive amount of meat, white bread and dairy products, are overweight and don't exercise much then you're in trouble. Furthermore if it's well-cooked red meat you like, which contains cancer promoting heterocyclic amines, and you consume reasonable amounts of mayonnaise, margarine and creamy salad dressings then you need to modify your eating habits. Along with meat and dairy products these foods increase the type of fats that raise testosterone and IGF-1 levels and promote inflammation, which is the kind of cocktail cancer cells thrive on.

Dairy, either in full-fat or skim-milk form, supplies both calcium and oestrogen and while calcium lowers protective vitamin D, the build-up of excessive oestrogen has already been identified as the prostate's principal enemy. (94) (95) The more milk you consume the greater the risk so that if you exceed two glasses per day the risk increases significantly. (96) White bread has a high glycaemic index, which provides cancer cells with all the sugar they need to grow.

Obesity and insulin resistance, the metabolic disorder it generates, are also highly unfavourable as these factors lead to more aggressive cancers that manifest at a younger age. If you gain weight rapidly in adulthood this can be especially dangerous as your body will be exposed to increasing amounts of oestrogen, insulin and IGF-1 which is a perfect hormonal platform for the development of prostate cancer. It stands to reason that a lack of exercise is going to set you up to put on weight, which will place you in just the metabolic zone that could lead to a disaster.

Two nutrients that you also need to be wary of are beta-carotene, which is preformed vitamin A, and zinc. While zinc has been shown to inhibit prostate cancer cells, there is evidence that zinc supplementation in the order of 100mg daily, which is a considerable amount of this nutrient, is associated with an increased risk of advanced prostate cancer. (96) The cause of this unexpected result is unknown but it may be related to zinc's capacity to increase testosterone, promote telomerase, an enzyme, which stimulates cancer cell growth and to zinc's ability to suppress the immune system in high doses. This tells us that you need to treat zinc with a lot of respect. If you are going to take zinc the 30mg limit should be observed which would be the equivalent of two zinc tablets daily.

Some studies show that beta-carotene is protective while others reveal exactly the opposite. One trial which did demonstrate the downside of beta-carotene supplementation was conducted on a group of Finnish smokers some years ago indicating that this nutrient lead to a slightly increased risk of developing prostate cancer. (97) There are those experts who claim that this had more to do with the adverse effects of cigarette smoking on the nature of beta-carotene and that smoking and vitamin supplementation are not exactly a marriage made in heaven. Current wisdom suggests that vitamin supplements should also be taken in combination rather than in an isolated fashion. Still caution should be observed when utilising beta-carotene.

ASSORTED TOXINS

ALCOHOL

Although there are studies which show that alcohol consumption does not harm the prostate, a Canadian study reviewing lifelong exposure found that regular drinking did increase the risk of developing prostate cancer and this became even more pronounced with daily use beginning before the age of 15. (98) An American study, which followed the drinking habits of Harvard alumni, similarly revealed that frequent consumers of alcohol suffered from a significantly increased incidence of prostate cancer. (99) Alcohol contains a number of substances that have been shown to be carcinogenic including ethanol, nitrosamines and acetaldehyde. The connection between raised IGF-1 levels and prostate cancer has already been established and there is a study which suggests that increasing alcohol intake boosts IGF-1 production. Alcohol also turns on the aromatase enzyme, which leads to heightened oestrogen exposure, another risk factor for developing cancer.

I'm not a great fan of habitual drinking and the implication that this kind of behaviour raises the odds for the development of prostate cancer indicates that safer activities should be substituted for this type of pastime. There are so many other enjoyable beverages out there such as grape juice, which is just as beneficial without the alcoholic toxins, or the vast array of herbal teas and assorted juices that it can't be that difficult to find a replacement.

PESTICIDES

Pesticides are bad news. They can act like hormones having the same effects that oestrogen and testosterone have on your prostate. However you don't have to be professionally associated with these chemicals to be affected. A recent pilot study conducted in Iowa intimates that long-term, low-dose exposure might be enough to increase your chances. (100)

This is a replica of the alcohol story except this time the danger lies in the simple daily pleasure of eating fruits and vegetables that are contaminated with pesticides. You only have to compare the taste of organic fruit and vegetables with the bland, vacuous quality of standard supermarket fare to realise that you are getting a product that is vastly more nutritious if it's organically grown. Although it's not always easy to follow this practice on a daily basis and it is more expensive, if you do have access to organic produce then treat yourself. You might just be doing your prostate a huge service.

HEAVY METALS

There aren't a whole lot of studies in this area but one carried out a long time ago demonstrated that if you inject rats daily for one month with lead and cadmium they will develop precancerous changes in their prostate. This doesn't necessarily mean that these substances cause cancer in humans but it does suggest that they are dangerous. If you want to discover whether your cells are being exposed to excessive amounts of heavy metals then you need to have a hair mineral analysis, which will give you a reasonable estimate of the accumulation of these toxins in your body.

ELECTROMAGNETIC RADIATION

Exposure to electromagnetic radiation is an occupational hazard rather than an everyday concern. Airline pilots and electric utility workers who experience more of this type of energy through their work situation have a higher risk of developing prostate cancer. A study which investigated the health problems of airline pilots over 17 years, found a connection between the number of long distance flights that they undertook and a rise in the incidence of prostate cancer. (101) This risk is possibly due to the electromagnetic fields from cockpit instruments that these pilots experience. Anyone involved in this type of work needs to pay added attention to the means for preventing prostate cancer which will be reviewed shortly.

INFLAMMATION

Inflammation is the essential driving force behind the development of prostate cancer. We already know that oestrogen stimulates inflammation which provokes free radical stress that damages DNA and this is how cancer cells are conceived. Aside from the overabundance of oestrogen there are other events which have the ability to fan the flames of inflammation. Red meat, especially the variety that is cooked at high temperature on charcoal grills, saturated fat found in substances like dairy products, and sexually transmitted infections such as the kind resulting from repeated exposure to gonorrhoea and syphilis also have the capacity to trigger inflammation which sets the cancer wheels in motion. The highly selected C-reactive protein (HS-CRP) blood test is one way to assess whether you are harbouring the seeds of inflammation in your body. An elevated HS-CRP indicates that inflammation is setting in and you need to take the appropriate measures to neutralise its presence before it gets the better of you. The medical way to do this is with drugs like aspirin and celebrex. These pharmaceuticals are not without their side effects and my preference is to opt for herbs like ginger and curcumin, which reduce inflammation without any negative consequences. Of course the most prudent strategy is to limit inflammation in the first place by restricting your consumption of red meat and diary products and adopting safe sex practices which minimise your contact with sexually transmitted nasties.

THE GENES

Age, race and a genetic predisposition are undoubtedly part of the story but it's also about the types of stresses that your prostate gland is exposed to which encompasses all the factors I've already mentioned. However, if you have a father or a brother who contracted this disease particularly at an earlier age, or your mother or sister has had breast cancer then your risk increases and you need to be more watchful. One of the ways you can do this is by having a regular PSA blood test and a good time to commence this process would be from the age of 50.

THE PSA

Until quite recently prostate cancer was diagnosed by means of an internal assessment of the prostate otherwise known as the digital rectal examination (DRE), an experience that is not eagerly anticipated by most men. It was sometimes discovered coincidentally when the prostate was operated on to relieve obstructive symptoms, such as the need to urinate often during the day and at night, caused by an enlarged prostate, a rather common experience for the ageing male. Oftentimes in these cases the diagnosis was made long after the cancer had spread beyond the prostate, which made it impossible to cure this rather insidious disease. It was only in 1987 that a seminal paper was released, which highlighted the exciting possibility of diagnosing prostate cancer by means of a simple blood test long before the cancer had begun to proliferate. So the much-heralded PSA (prostate specific antigen), which promised to offer a unique means for diagnosing prostate cancer, (there was no equivalent test to identify breast, bowel cancer or indeed the cancer of any other organ) assumed a lofty position on the world stage.

The PSA is a protein which adds to the fluid of the ejaculate making this vital secretion more mobile and therefore more capable of reaching the awaiting eggs. A damaged prostate releases more PSA into the bloodstream and it was found that excess levels of this substance were increasingly associated with the presence of prostate cancer. The problem is that a raised PSA is not a 100% diagnostic of prostate cancer. This kind of result might simply mean your prostate is enlarged. It can even go up if you've ejaculated the night before you have a test or if your prostate is inflamed. In 25% of cases you might have prostate cancer and have what is considered to be a normal PSA reading. We used to think that the cut-off point for concern was 4ng/ml. If your PSA was below this score then you could breathe easy about the health of your prostate.

That was until the release of a report in the New England Journal of Medicine May 2004, which investigated the prevalence of prostate cancer in 18,882 men enrolled in the Prostate Cancer prevention trial and found, much to everyone's dismay, that the incidence of cancer was not rare among men with a PSA score less than 4ng/ml. (102) There were even those with a PSA less than 0.5ng/ml who had cancer. Because of these findings an utterly safe score is now thought to be a miserly 0.25ng/ml.

What is also becoming more utilised these days are a number of other prognostic features generated by the PSA test. (103) One of these is the free/total PSA ratio. PSA is located in the bloodstream either in free form or attached to a protein. It has been found that cancer sufferers have more of the attached variety indicating that less free PSA increases the likelihood of a positive diagnosis. The lower the ratio of free to total PSA the greater is the risk of having prostate cancer. For those with a PSA score between 4-10ng/ml and a ratio of less than 0.1 the chances of having cancer are 56% while these decrease to 8% with a ratio of more than 0.25. The other measure that is gaining popularity is the PSA velocity or the PSA doubling time and this looks at the degree to which the PSA increases over time. If your PSA increases by more than 0.75ng/ml over the space of a year or your calculated doubling time is rather rapid then this is thought to indicate that something suspicious is afoot and further investigations such as an ultrasound scan, which might even lead to a biopsy, should be considered.

You probably have a reasonable sense by now that the PSA is no godsend. As a result of all these complexities as well as the recent findings and previous concerns about the lack of specificity of the PSA with regard to diagnosing prostate cancer, this test is now bathed in a sea of controversy with little universal agreement about its usefulness as a screening tool. There are those experts who claim that you should have your PSA measured annually from the age of 50 together with an internal evaluation of your prostate by means of the good old digital examination. This might lead to early detection of cancer and curative treatment before the horse has bolted. There are others who claim that an elevated PSA score might lead to unnecessary worry and procedures such as biopsies, which have their own complications, merely to discover that you probably don't have prostate cancer. Yet the lingering doubt might remain.

I have no easy answer for this accept to mention the case of Barry, a delightful gentleman in his late fifties who had never had a PSA test, but was prompted to have this investigation by his much younger wife who was concerned about the fact that he was going to the toilet rather often especially at night. She had just seen a programme about prostate cancer on television. Barry wasn't totally unconcerned about his health. He did take multivitamins, had a reasonable diet which included regular servings of fish and steamed vegetables, but he did enjoy his alcohol, sometimes to the extent of drinking six beers a night, and he was overweight.

Barry's PSA score was 5ng/ml and his free/total ratio was 0.2, which did raise the alarm bells and an HS-CRP score of 50 suggesting a significant degree of inflammation wasn't very reassuring either. The surgeon suggested that Barry have an immediate biopsy and needless to say a positive cancer diagnosis was the outcome. If there is an upside to all of this it's the possibility that an operation and the removal of Barry's prostate (which is not without its own complications) can be totally curative whereas had Barry not had this timely test the cancer might have spread and troubled him at a time when it had become utterly lethal.

Barry's predicament leads me to believe that regular screening and early detection of cancer is worthwhile. What you actually do with an elevated PSA score, that could mean any number of things, has unfortunately to be evaluated each time on its merits. You can also choose not to have a regular PSA test. However I would still advise an annual DRE after the age of fifty and a medical assessment if you are having symptoms which suggest your prostate is compromised, such as a weakening stream or the need to go to the men's room often during the day and frequently at night. My major priority though is with prevention and before we proceed to elaborate on the further steps you can take to minimise your chances of succumbing to this disease it would be worthwhile revising all the risk factors for prostate cancer.

Risk factors for prostate cancer

- Elevated oestrogen levels especially the 2 hydroxyoestrogens and the 3,4 quinone oestrogens
- Raised testosterone and dihydrotestosterone levels
- High levels of IGF-1
- Inflammation
- Free radical stress
- Vitamin D deficiency and excess
- Ageing
- Being of African-American extraction
- Living in North America and North-western Europe
- Red meat
- Dairy products
- Saturated fat
- Obesity
- Insulin resistance
- Excessive zinc supplementation
- Regular and excessive alcohol consumption
- Pesticides
- Lead
- Cadmium
- Family history and a genetic predisposition
- Raised PSA

PREVENTING PROSTATE CANCER

THE HORMONES

Prostate cancer can take up to twenty years before it rears its ugly head and even then you may not even know that you have cancer until you have an operation to deal with the symptoms that result from an enlarged prostate. A good plan of action would be to see to it that your hormones are well balanced so that your prostate is not exposed to excessive amounts of either testosterone, oestrogen or dihydrotestosterone. If you eliminate testosterone you probably won't get prostate cancer but no man would be happy to function without this vital hormone. What you need to ensure is that your levels don't go much higher than 30nmol/Litre especially if you are taking testosterone or augmenting your body's production of this hormone if your levels are low.

Resveratrol, the red grape extract, which possesses a multitude of anti-cancer properties, can prevent testosterone from having an overly stimulating effect on your prostate. The herb saw palmetto, which has been shown to effectively treat prostatic enlargement, can also temper any testosterone that has become overactive. What this herb also does is to inhibit the enzyme 5 alpha-reductase, which converts testosterone to dihydrotestosterone. This would equally be beneficial if your dihydrotestosterone levels are too high which can be established with a blood test.

Japanese men have the lowest incidence of prostate cancer in the world and this might be attributed to significant findings in the early 1990's which indicated that this group of men have substantially lower levels of 5 alpha-reductase in their prostates when compared with white and black men from the United States. Other natural substances, which act on 5 alpha-reductase, are zinc and the phyto-oestrogens found in soy, red clover and flaxseed. Remember with zinc you don't want to go beyond 30mg per day, which is usually two zinc tablets, if you supplement with this mineral, as the study reported earlier did show that taking 100mg daily is associated with an increased risk of developing prostate cancer.

Aside from modulating 5-alpha reductase, saw palmetto also has anti-inflammatory effects, inhibits those cells, which promote cancer growth and gets in the way of IGF-1, the cancer cell stimulator. A recent clinical trial has demonstrated that the medication finasteride (otherwise known as proscar) used to treat enlargement of the prostate also has the power to prevent prostate cancer. (104) The one problem that did occur in this impressive experiment was that although the group of men taking this medication experienced a significantly lower cancer incidence than the placebo group there was a higher rate of more aggressive cancers in the treatment group. Experts have been scrambling to explain this rather baffling finding which undermined the enthusiasm greeting the outcome of this trial.

The good or bad news about these findings is that finasteride by inhibiting 5 alpha-reductase operates in pretty much the same fashion as saw palmetto. The one advantage that saw palmetto does have over finasteride is that 5 alpha-reductase is composed of two isoenzymes and while finasteride predominantly targets the type 2 form the action of saw palmetto encompasses both isoenzymes. The other major bonus that saw palmetto brings to the equation is that unlike finasteride this herb does not lower your PSA which is useful if you want to periodically assess the status of your prostate by means of a regular blood test. Therefore we can surmise that taking saw palmetto for an extended period of time because of its protective effects might be more beneficial as well as safer than finasteride without any negative spin-offs. However, without long-term trials all we can do is speculate. With all its many benefits I'm going to side with saw palmetto. A good dose of saw palmetto would be 160mg twice daily.

The other piece in the jigsaw is to keep control of oestrogen. Men do need oestrogen. It's good for our bones, helps with our sexual function and probably contributes in some way to preventing Alzheimer's. The problem is that having too much of it is bad for our prostate. There's a politically tricky joke about knowing when you have too much oestrogen, which is the time you find you want to go shopping for no obvious reason or you enter into incessant conversation with no particular goal in mind or you allow your partner to dominate the remote control without a squabble. Oh, the many joys of oestrogen. The other way is to pay attention to any relentless gain in weight and the development of those unsightly 'maleboobs' as fat cells possess the enzyme aromatase, which increases your oestrogen levels. Having more than two cups of coffee per day or exceeding your daily limit of two alcoholic drinks will also stimulate aromatase. Aromatase inhibitors include resveratrol, soy, flaxseed, red clover and quercetin.

A poorly functioning liver will also increase oestrogen as will tight fitting underwear of all things. The cells of your testes secrete testosterone and oestrogen and believe it or not undergarments that cling to your scrotum compromise your blood supply which favours oestrogen.

Once your oestrogen levels exceed 110pmol/Litre then you are starting to exceed healthy limits. Another useful test to have is to measure your levels of 2 and 16 hydroxyoestrogens by means of a urine test. The 2 hyroxyoestrogens are the healthier variety and you need double the quantity of these hormones compared with the 16 hydoxyoestrogens to achieve an optimal ratio.

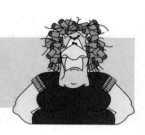

To much oestrogen is bad
for your prostate

THE VITAMINS

Of all the trials which have examined the effects of vitamin supplementation on the prevention of prostate cancer, vitamin E is the one nutrient that emerges with real potential to prevent this disease. Vitamin E is comprised of various isoforms including alpha-, beta-, gamma- and delta-tocopherols as well as the tocotrienols. This nutrient is found in nuts, seeds, soybeans, wheat germ, vegetables oils such as safflower, sunflower, cottonseed, canola and olive oils together with palm, rice bran and coconut oils. While gamma-tocopherol is the predominant form of vitamin E in the diet, alpha-tocopherol is found in much higher quantities in the bloodstream. Vitamin E is a powerful antioxidant with alpha and gamma-tocopherol having complimentary roles in neutralising highly toxic free radicals.

One study has demonstrated that supplementing with 50mg of alpha-tocopherol reduced the incidence of prostate cancer in a group of Finnish smokers by 32% while another indicated that high levels of gamma-tocopherol in the bloodstream lead to a hefty 81% decline in prostate cancer incidence. (105) (106) Unless you're an avid consumer of nuts, seeds and oils you're unlikely to enjoy the protective benefits of vitamin E. A healthy supplementary dose of this vitamin would be 200-400mg of mixed tocopherols with 50mg of combination tocotrienols.

THE DIET AND EXERCISE

The incidence of prostate cancer in Japan is approximately one-tenth of that in the United States. Conversely the rate of prostate cancer amongst Japanese immigrants in Hawaii is ten times that of the homeland. Diet probably has a whole lot to do with this as the traditional Japanese diet, which consists mostly of fish and soybean products including tofu, miso and natto (fermented soybeans), is associated with a decreased risk of prostate cancer while the saturated fat rich western diet with lots of meat and dairy products promotes cancer.

If you can adjust your taste buds to the delights of fish and soybeans then you can add the brassica family to your plate, as nutrient-dense vegetables such as cabbage, cauliflower, broccoli, Brussels sprouts, kale and kohlrabi have been shown to be protective in some studies. (107) The benefits of exercise with regard to prostate cancer haven't been explored but it stands to reason that if you exercise regularly and keep your weight down you won't have all that extra cancer promoting oestrogen floating around.

THE SPECIAL NUTRIENTS

SOY

In the Asian diet one of the principle substances that contributes to the low incidence of prostate cancer is thought to be soy. One Japanese study has shown that high levels of the metabolites of soy in the bloodstream lead to a lower incidence of prostate cancer. (108) In a study, which evaluated the protective habits of Seventh-Day Adventists in California, those men who consumed soymilk more than once a day experienced a 70% reduction in the risk of prostate cancer. (109)

By increasing the carrier protein, sex hormone binding globulin that transports testosterone and oestrogen around the body, soy is able to reduce the stimulatory effects that these hormones have on the prostate. Soy also operates by getting in the way of the initiation phase of tumour development and if this isn't enough soy also inhibits the cancer cell cycle, reduces inflammation and then for good measure cuts off the blood supply to any cancer cells that have escaped this surveillance operation.

If you haven't acquired a taste for soy or tofu, tempeh, which blends quite nicely into a stir fry, and miso, then you can try eating more peas, beans and lentils as these will provide you with comparable amounts of genistein and daidzein, the major end-products of soy in the bloodstream. Despite the roller-coaster ride that soy has endured, the one minute it's good for you the next minute it's not, there appears to be sound evidence here that this substance and its metabolites will help to protect your prostate.

LYCOPENE

Lycopene is the pigment which gives the tomato its red colour. This substance is also found in guava, apricots and watermelon. Lycopene is a powerful antioxidant and its job is to protect the fruit where it resides against the toxic effects of oxygen and light. There is some evidence that high levels of this substance in the bloodstream might have a similar impact on the prevention of prostate cancer. (110) Lycopene is much better absorbed from processed tomato products such as tomato sauce. There is also evidence which seems to suggest that it is a complex array of nutrients found in substances like tomato sauce or tomatoes combined with oils such as olive oil rather than lycopene alone which provide the most protective benefits. (111)

A test tube study has shown that lycopene on its own was not able to prevent the build-up of prostate cancer cells, however, when this substance was combined with vitamin E there was a considerable reduction in tumour growth. Like they do in the natural environment nutrients always function optimally when used in combination. While encouraging you to consume lycopene rich fruits especially tomatoes cooked with a hint of olive oil in a stir fry that will make this nutrient more readily absorbable my advice is also to supplement with lycopene. Studies show that consuming between 5-10 serves of tomatoes and tomato-based products is what you need to provide you with some protection. To this I would suggest you add 5-10 mg of lycopene.

SELENIUM

Selenium is found in Brazil nuts, broccoli, cabbages, onions, garlic, grains, fish, meat, eggs and dairy. The amount of selenium in food depends on the selenium content of soil. This nutrient enters the food chain through plants and as certain areas of the world are depleted of selenium this has negative ramifications for the health of the prostate. Selenium forms an essential component of the glutathione antioxidant system, which is responsible for eliminating toxins and protecting against DNA damage. Selenium also enhances the immune system and there is good evidence that this nutrient operates to kill off cancer cells and to prevent them from establishing themselves in the body at the early stages of cancer development. Like many other anti-cancer agents selenium also encourages cancer cells to commit suicide, prevents them from multiplying and cuts off their blood supply.

There are a number of studies indicating that elevated concentrations of selenium reduce the risk of prostate cancer.

(110) Interestingly one study has demonstrated that high selenium levels only became protective when they were associated with raised levels of gamma tocopherol, which forms part of vitamin E, indicating once again that nutrients function optimally in tandem. (111) Another study has revealed that supplementing with 200micrograms of selenium significantly reduced the incidence of prostate cancer especially in those men who had low levels of this nutrient. (112) If you want to establish where your selenium levels are at then you need to have a blood test, which measures your white blood cell selenium content. My suggestion is that you supplement with 200micrograms per day anyway particularly if your levels are low.

FISH OIL

Fish oils are rich in omega-3 fatty acids, which are metabolised to eicosapentanoic acid (EPA) and docosahexanoic acid (DHA). These are powerful anti-inflammatory agents and it is their ability to counteract the pro-inflammatory forces found in the omega-6 containing margarines and vegetable oils, which probably contributes to their cancer inhibiting effects. Studies, which have examined the fish consuming habits of various nations, seem to indicate that it is the cold water fish such as salmon, mackerel, sardines and herring which have the highest concentrations of EPA and DHA that offer the most protection. (113) This was confirmed by New Zealand research showing that elevated levels of red blood cell EPA and DHA considerably reduced prostate cancer risk. American natural health experts Dr Michael Murray and Dr Joseph Pizzorno in the highly informative book ' How to Prevent and Treat Cancer with Natural Medicine' recommend at least two servings of cold-water fish per week and it would be wise to go for the smaller fish to reduce the chances of mercury contamination. In addition to which they suggest you should also take 120-360mg of EPA and 80-240mg of DHA, especially if you are at risk.

FLAXSEED

Unfortunately there aren't any studies which have examined the protective effects of flaxseed with regard to the development of prostate cancer. However, this nutrient does have the potential to reduce oestrogen and testosterone levels, which would make it a useful substance to take especially if your oestrogen levels are elevated. The best way to benefit from flaxseed is in its ground form combined with crushed almonds and sunflower seeds in what is known as the LSA (linseed, sunflower seeds and almonds) mix. Two tablespoons would be a reasonable daily dose and you can sprinkle those over your breakfast cereal or a yoghurt and fruit combination.

INDOLE-3 CARBINOL AND DIINDOLYLMETHANE

3,3 Diindolylmethane (DIM) is a major digestive product of indole-3-carbinol and both of these substance are found in cruciferous vegetables such as broccoli, Brussels sprouts, kale and cauliflower, the consumption of which has been shown to reduce the incidence of prostate cancer. Test tube studies have demonstrated that these nutrients have the ability to suppress cancer cell growth. They also have the power to increase the ratio of 2 to 16 hydroxyoestrogens and to inhibit the formation of 4-hydroxyoestrogens, which make indole-3-carbinol and diindolylmethane ideal candidates for prostate cancer prevention. (114) (115) If you don't enjoy the taste of cruciferous vegetables and adding hummus, tahini or pesto don't make these vegetables any more palatable then it would be a good idea to consider supplementation. A good dose of indole-3 carbinol would be 150mg twice daily while that of diindolylmethane would be 260mg also taken twice a day.

GREEN TEA

There is evidence that regular consumers of tea have a lower risk of prostate cancer-related deaths. (116) Green tea and black tea are derived from the same source, the difference being that black tea leaves undergo extensive fermentation, which reduces their antioxidant content. This makes green tea much more protective which would imply that drinking this form of tea would be a sounder investment. 2-4 cups per day would offer you some added protection against prostate cancer.

RESVERATROL

I know I've mentioned this nutrient before in this section but I'm so impressed by the promise of resveratrol to prevent prostate cancer that I really do believe it should occupy a premier position in everyone's preventive strategy. Resveratrol has the ability to inhibit the initiation stage of cancer development as well as every phase of cancer cell growth. There is also evidence that at high concentrations resveratrol combined with genistein found in soy operate very effectively to stop cancer cell progression. (117) Resveratrol is found in grape skins and while red wine consumption has its benefits the wine making process leads to the elimination of this critical nutrient. You could try drinking grape juice but I'm also going to advise that you supplement with 5-20mg of resveratrol daily.

QUERCETIN

This is another protective nutrient that you can keep up your sleeve. Quercetin is a bioflavonoid, (a vitamin-like substance) found in onions and apples as well as citrus fruits, tea, grapes, red wine, parsley, olive oil, dark cherries, and dark berries, such as blueberries, blackberries, and bilberries, that has antioxidant, immune boosting and anti-cancer potential. This is in addition to quercetin's ability to lower oestrogen levels by restricting the activity of the enzyme aromatase. A healthy protective dose of quercetin would be 500-1000mg daily.

VITAMIN D

Vitamin D can be obtained from enriched dairy products, fish oils and eggs or you can simply spend 20 minutes in the direct sunlight to get your daily dose of fortification. With all its abilities to inhibit cancer cells in so many different ways it would be foolhardy not to see to it that you are getting your protective dose of 1000i.u.s daily.

Here then is a list of all the herbs and nutrients you can incorporate to prevent prostate cancer. While none of these will guarantee 100% protection it is really the combination of these substances that offers the most cover.

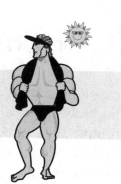

All you need is
20 Minutes in the Sun

What prevents prostate cancer

- Saw palmetto 160mg twice daily
- Vitamin E consisting of mixed tocopherols 200-400mg daily
- Vitamin E consisting of mixed tocotrienols 50mg daily
- Vitamin B12 500micrograms daily
- Folic acid 500micrograms daily
- Alpha-lipoic acid 200mg daily
- Soybean products including miso, tofu and natto
- Cruciferous vegetables found in broccoli, Brussels sprouts, cabbage and cauliflower
- Lycopene 10-20mg daily
- Selenium 200micrograms daily
- Fish oils containing 120-360mg of EPA and 80-240mg of DHA daily
- Flaxseed 2 tablespoons daily
- Indole-3 carbinol 150mg twice daily or Diindolylmethane 260mg twice daily
- Green tea 2-4 cups daily
- Resveratrol 5-20mg daily
- Quercetin 500-1000mg daily
- Vitamin D 1000i.u. daily

TREATING PROSTATE CANCER

Remember David? He was the unfortunate gentleman in his early fifties whose prostate cancer was diagnosed after a routine PSA test. Fortunately the biopsy revealed that his tumour would probably respond favourably to surgery or radiotherapy. Sadly some cancers are more aggressive and grow more rapidly rendering these types of therapies less effective. In this scenario hormone treatments, which antagonise the stimulating effects of testosterone and dihydrotestosterone, are used. Although David's prognosis was a good one he still wanted to augment his treatment with dietary strategies and natural therapies that might improve his outcome. Here's what's available to David with our current state of knowledge.

THE HORMONES

There is encouraging evidence that just as melatonin has a favourable effect on breast cancer this hormone might equally have a significant impact on prostate cancer. Test tube studies show that melatonin has the ability to inhibit cancer cell growth. (118) Hormone treatment for prostate cancer is designed to suppress testosterone. Difficulties arise when a certain group of cancer cells take evasive action and find a way to thrive independently of hormonal stimulation, which makes conventional treatment rather ineffectual.

Exciting evidence indicates that melatonin might just offer alternative possibilities. Two studies, one on an individual patient and another on a group of cancer sufferers have shown that melatonin, at a dose of 5mg daily in the case of the lone patient and 20mg daily in the case of the larger group found a way to outsmart the cancer cells and significantly improved the prognosis of those taking this hormone. (119) (120) I usually start patients off on a 5mg dose of melatonin taken at night as this hormone might lead to daytime drowsiness if the initial dose is too high. If this is well tolerated then this treatment can be advanced gradually to 20mg.

VITAMINS AND ANTIOXIDANTS

Aside from melatonin the combination of vitamins C and E has been shown to put an end to cancer cells. In a similar fashion the teamwork of vitamin E and lycopene has been shown to be equally effective. Vitamin E and selenium display a similar synergy. To get the full benefit from vitamin E you need to incorporate all the tocopherols and tocotrienols as these all have some part to play in eradicating cancer cells.

Vitamin C needs to be taken in high doses with 5-10grams daily being a respectable dose. The daily dose of vitamin E would be 200-400mg per day of the mixed tocopherols together with 50mg of the combined tocotrienols.

There are a number of animal and cell culture studies showing that cancer cells are exquisitely sensitive to vitamin D. This vitamin encourages cancer cells to mutate into normal cells and it also coerces prostate cancer cells into committing suicide. Any wayward cancer cells that have escaped the clutches of vitamin D are prevented from spreading beyond the prostate once this vitamin gets its ever-expanding tentacles on these cells. A reasonable starting dose of vitamin D would be 3000-5000i.u.daily

In addition to teaming up with vitamin E, lycopene or at least a tomato-rich concentrate containing this nutrient has been shown to reduce the PSA and improve the outcome in a group of men about to have a prostatectomy. (121) For those men taking lycopene their cancers had shrunk by the time the operation came about and there was also less damage to the tissue surrounding the cancer once the operation was completed. 5-20mg of lycopene daily would provide a therapeutic dose.

Aside from the multitalented resveratrol, which has the ability to inhibit cancer cells, quercetin has been shown to have remarkably similar talents. In cell culture studies quercetin was able to check the growth of prostate cancer cells especially those with the most aggressive intent. The biggest problem with cancer cells is that they have the potential to become immortal with the ability to replicate forever. What quercetin does is to outwit cancer cells by deftly switching on tumour suppressor genes, which stop cancer cells dead in their tracks. While resveratrol should be administered at a dose of 5-20mg daily a reasonable dose of quercetin would be 500-1000mg daily.

The real point about vitamins is that they operate more effectively in combination just like in nature where fruits and vegetables harbour a multitude of beneficial nutrients. I would really encourage supplementation with all these nutrients in the doses indicated rather than individually and in smaller doses

HERBAL MEDICINES AND OTHER REMEDIES

The advantage of herbal medicines is that they often augment conventional treatments, making side-effects more endurable and introducing the option of reducing the dose of chemotherapeutic agents, which are often highly toxic to normal cells. Not only do they directly target cancer cells but they also operate by boosting the immune system and the body's natural recuperative powers thereby enhancing survival possibilities.

Green tea, silibinin, the active component of the herb st mary's thistle, curcumin, the major yellow pigment extracted from tumeric which is used to spice curries, saw palmetto and astragalus, the immune boosting herb, all have the ability to terminate prostate cancer cells and prevent them from spreading. These natural therapies also have the potential to treat cancers that are no longer sensitive to conventional treatments, which might offer some tangible hope to those cancer sufferers who aren't winning the battle with hormonal interventions and chemotherapy.

Six cups a day would give you a reasonable amount of green tea but if you find this difficult taking two capsules daily each containing 125mg of green tea extract would also provide you with a healthy dose of this herb. 250mg of silibinin, which is thought to be the most biologically active component of st mary's thistle, would equip you with a therapeutic dose of this substance. The dose of curcumin is somewhere between 200-400mg taken in either capsule or tablet form one to three times daily. The best way to absorb curcumin is to ingest this substance on an empty stomach 20 minutes before meals. The dose of astragalus is 8-10grams daily while that of saw palmetto is 160mg taken twice daily.

Studies show that indole-3 carbinol and diindolylmethane have the ability to inhibit cancer cells. Modified citrus pectin, which is derived from the skins of citrus fruit, can be used to prevent cancer cells from spreading. Inositol hexaphosphate (Ip6), which is found in cereals, nuts, legumes, seeds and soybeans is another substance which is able to suppress cancer cells. The substantial presence of Ip6 in the Asian diet might be another reason that the incidence of prostate cancer is much lower in Asian countries compared with Western countries. PSK is a substance derived from a mushroom called Coriolus versicolor that contains a powerful immune-boosting nutrient called beta-glucans which is also found in Maitake D-fraction extract. Like modified citrus pectin PSK has the potential to restrict metastatic spread of prostate cancer.

A therapeutic dose of indole-3 carbinol would be 300mg twice daily and that of diindolylmethane 520mg twice daily. The recommended daily dosage for modified citrus pectin is 20-30 grams. Murray and Pizzorno recommend 4800-7200mg of Ip6 together with 1200-1800mg of inositol and suggest that this be taken on an empty stomach. 1-3 grams per day would be the usual dose of PSK.

As is the case with vitamin and antioxidant therapy the combination of these remedies would have a far greater impact on cancer growth than using each one of these on its own.

DIET

The prostate cancer-friendly diet is pretty much the same as the one suggested for the management of breast cancer. If you can you should avoid red meat and dairy products and your diet should be comprised mostly of vegetables, wholegrain breads and cereals, fruits, some fish and eggs with an emphasis on the green vegetables such as broccoli, spinach, rocket, cabbage and cauliflower. Maintaining your ideal weight and limiting your consumption of alcohol and refined carbohydrates such as candy bars, chocolates, cakes and ice-cream would be a good idea. Regular exercise would also be beneficial.

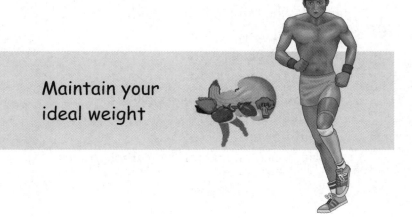

Maintain your
ideal weight

Treating prostate cancer

- Melatonin 5-20mg daily
- Vitamin C 5-10 grams daily
- Vitamin E mixed tocopherols 200-400mg daily
- Vitamin E mixed tocotrienols 50mg daily
- Vitamin D 3000-5000 i.u.daily
- Lycopene 5-20mg daily
- Resveratrol 5-20mg daily
- Quercetin 500-1000mg daily
- Green tea 6 cups or 250mg daily
- Silibinin 250mg daily
- Curcumin 200-400mg one to three times daily
- Astragalus 8-10 grams daily
- Saw palmetto 160mg daily
- Indole-3 carbinol 300mg twice daily or diindolylmethane 520mg twice daily
- Modified citrus Pectin 20-30grams daily
- Ip6 4800-7200 mg plus 1200-1800mg of inositol daily
- PSK 13 grams daily
- Avoid red meat and dairy products
- Eat lots of cruciferous vegetables including spinach, broccoli, cabbage and cauliflower
- Limit alcohol and refined carbohydrates

COLORECTAL CANCER

Colorectal cancer (CRC), which encompasses all cancers of the large bowel, is a significant health concern affecting nearly 150,000 people in the USA every year with close to 60,000 deaths expected in 2004. This is a rather depressing statistic seeing that CRC, which develops over 10-20 years allowing for all the appropriate anticipatory measures, is so eminently preventable.

RISK FACTORS FOR COLORECTAL CANCER

THE HORMONES

CRC is the third leading cause of cancer deaths in women and this may have a lot to do with the absence of the protective effects of oestrogen. The risk of developing CRC increases with ageing when oestrogen production dwindles. There is also evidence that women with lower bone mass, which is thought to depend on the presence of oestrogen, are more vulnerable to developing CRC. Add to this all those studies including the recent Women's Health Initiative trial, which show that HRT in the form of oestrogen alone or in combination with progestins leads to a lower incidence of CRC, and there is persuasive evidence that enhancing oestrogen levels might at least be part of the female defensive strategy for preventing CRC. Women have one over men here because testosterone doesn't appear to provide any protective benefits.

The other hormone that features in the picture is melatonin. A study that followed rotating night-shift workers over a 15-year period found that working such a shift for at least three nights per month over this time led to a greater incidence of CRC and this might be related to a substantial reduction in melatonin production. (122) Melatonin is produced at night when you sleep and if you expose your body to light, which is what shift-workers have to do, melatonin levels will go down. If you are on such a work schedule or you want to find out whether your body is producing enough melatonin then you need to have your levels tested via a nighttime salivary sample. Once you discover that your levels are low then extra melatonin might be beneficial and you can start off with 1mg taken at night, which you can increase to 3mg. Foods such as soy products, almonds, tomatoes and wild rice also have the potential to increase your natural production of melatonin.

VITAMIN DEFICIENCIES

Folic acid is vitally important for the formation of healthy DNA and there is a lot of evidence which connects low levels of this vitamin with the development of CRC. Low levels of vitamin B12 and methionine, an amino acid found in sunflower seeds, avocado and wild game which join forces with folic acid to build DNA, have also been linked to cancer development. In one American study low levels of beta-carotene, lycopene and vitamin E were all linked with an increased risk of rectal cancer in women especially those with low supplies of oestrogen. (122)

DIET AND WEIGHT GAIN

Red meat, especially the well-done variety, processed meats, refined carbohydrates found in biscuits, doughnuts, muffins and cookies, the fats in margarine, mayonnaise, salad oil and cooking oil, dairy, although this seems to be relevant only to certain racial groups such as African-Americans, and even an increased frequency of egg consumption, more than five per week for men and three for women, lead to a heightened risk of developing CRC. If you don't like vegetables you're also in a bit of strife as a lack of these in your daily diet also increases your vulnerability. Being overweight will add to your woes probably via that old nemesis insulin resistance.

ASSORTED TOXINS

ALCOHOL

There is almost universal agreement that regular alcohol consumption increases your risk with an even stronger association once your intake hits seven drinks per week. Those who have a passion for beer need to be aware of a study which has shown that daily beer consumers had a 12-fold elevated risk of sigmoid colon cancer compared with abstainers. Alcohol becomes even more harmful if you are deficient in vitamins A, C, E and folic acid with a Polish study indicating that those who have a higher consumption of alcohol have a noticeably magnified risk of developing CRC once these nutrients are on the low side. (123)

PESTICIDES

There is one Egyptian study which found that CRC patients had a high blood level of organochlorine pesticides. (124) It does make sense to eat as much pesticide-free food as you can get your hands on especially if you have other risk factors for the development of CRC.

BOWEL GERMS

The bowel is the home of millions of bacteria, which coexist in a complex ecosystem that contributes in a highly significant fashion to your overall health. Disturbances in this delicate balance can lead to serious health problems and possibly cancer. Even germs that normally function as commensals, which means they are usually harmless, have the potential to be lethal. One of these is the old enemy candida albicans, which might be dangerous in its own right or by virtue of the fact that it can produce excessive concentrations of acetaldehyde, a chemical with the ability to disrupt those proteins important for DNA repair. Although it's not totally clear how commensals can become agents that promote cancer, a lot might have to do with what you put in your mouth.

While a diet that is high in yeast and sugars encourages the growth of candida albicans, alcohol, as well as the heterocyclic amines found in well-cooked red meat, can combine with commensals to generate substances that can cause cancer. While you can watch your diet to ensure that you are limiting your consumption of these offending foods you can also have a urine test which will tell you whether you have an imbalance of germs in your bowel that are producing any damaging chemicals. This is the test which measures organic acids with abnormal levels of these being good indicators of bowel disharmony (see final chapter).

IRON

You might be wondering why an essential mineral is occupying a position in the toxins group. We can't do without iron as this mineral helps transmit oxygen around our bodies but too much iron can be harmful. High iron levels can lead to the accumulation of free radicals, which damage DNA. There is a hereditary condition known as hemochromatosis that is characterised by the excessive absorption of iron, which can incapacitate the liver, the heart, the pancreas and other organs. But it doesn't end there. In 2003 an American study investigated hemochromatosis gene mutations amongst colon cancer sufferers and found that subjects with any gene mutations were more likely to have cancer than those without any mutations. (125) The authors of this study also found that the association between colon cancer risk and these gene mutations intensified with ageing and a greater intake of iron. A gene mutation indicates that you can transmit this disease but you don't actually have hemochromatosis.

For the record, at least 20% of most white populations possess gene mutations for hemochromatosis. Why there is such a connection amongst those who don't even have hemochromatosis and the propensity to develop bowel cancer is a mystery for now and the authors of this study concede that these findings are preliminary and need substantiation in further testing.

Without wishing to set off the panic button there is a very simple way to discover whether you have an iron problem. All you need to do is have a blood test and if your iron levels are high then you need to proceed to a gene assay test. If this investigation does indicate that you have the gene and your iron levels are elevated then one way you can reduce your iron stores is by becoming a blood donor. Green tea, lactoferrin, which is found in whey protein, and the herb st mary's thistle have the ability to neutralise excess iron and you shouldn't take any vitamin C in supplementary form as this nutrient increases the absorption of iron.

INFLAMMATION

Inflammation is undoubtably a prime mover behind the development of CRC. Both Crohn's disease and ulcerative colitis, inflammatory conditions of the bowel, can lead to the development of CRC, however, with effective anti-inflammatory treatments this risk is considerably reduced. Aside from these inflammatory bowel conditions there are a host of other factors which promote inflammation including bowel infections, free radical stress and a lack of antioxidant protection. A British study has even linked obesity, physical inactivity and increasing age with the development of inflammation. (126)

A blood test which measures highly sensitive C-reactive protein (HS-CRP) can identify the presence of inflammation and American research has shown that this test can predict who will develop CRC. (127) In a study which followed a large group of individuals from 1989 till the year 2000 those who had an elevated HS-CRP had a significantly increased risk for subsequently developing cancer. Although this test is not specific for bowel inflammation it is a very simple investigation to have and if your levels are elevated then you can address all the underlying events that precipitate this condition as well as introduce all the strategies that reduce inflammation.

GENES

Having a first-degree relative with CRC especially someone who has had bowel cancer before the age of 50 results in a twofold increase in risk. However what the scientific evidence also tells us is that a healthy lifestyle and the appropriate dietary choices can considerably reduce this risk. A Hawaiian study has demonstrated that men with a family history of CRC who observed a healthy lifestyle did not experience an increased risk of developing cancer while those with an unhealthy lifestyle significantly increased their risk. (128) Simply eating more fruit, vegetables, grains, poultry and fish and moving away from a Western-style diet that is high in red meat, fast food and refined carbohydrates diminished the risk of developing CRC among those with a first-degree relative with CRC. This in addition to regular sigmoidoscopy screening is one of the most important factors that reduces the risk of CRC.

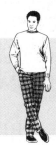

Beware of bad Genes

Risk factors for colorectal cancer

- Low oestrogen levels
- Low melatonin levels
- Folic acid deficiency
- Vitamin B12 deficiency
- Methionine deficiency
- Low levels of beta-carotene, lycopene and vitamin E
- Red meat, especially the well-done variety
- Refined carbohydrates

- The fats in margarine, mayonnaise, salad and cooking oil
- Excessive egg consumption
- High body mass
- Excessive alcohol consumption
- Pesticides
- Imbalance of bowel germs
- High iron levels associated with hemochromatosis and hemochromatosis gene mutations
- Inflammation and inflammatory bowel diseases
- A first-degree relative with CRC

PREVENTING CRC

THE HORMONES

Oestrogen is the foremost hormone with the ability to prevent CRC according to the WHI study, which showed that combined hormone replacement and oestrogen alone leads to a lower incidence of cancer in postmenopausal women. DHEA also demonstrates anti-tumor activity in an animal model, which raises the possibility that this might also be applicable to humans.

THE VITAMINS

Folic acid, vitamin D, vitamin C, vitamin E and beta-carotene are the nutrients that have been shown to have protective effects in some studies. The sooner you start taking vitamins the better. A study, which followed the progress of a large group of nurses found that those women who took folate-rich multivitamins for more than 14 years had a 75% reduction in CRC risk compared with non users. (129) The trick is also to supplement with just the right amount of folic acid, which would be around 400micrograms daily.

THE DIET AND WEIGHT GAIN

Despite a number of contradictory studies concerning the contribution of a high-fibre diet to the prevention of CRC there appears to be some agreement now that the daily consumption of raw fruit and vegetables will help to prevent CRC with cruciferous and green vegetables being the most protective. While you're enjoying your fruit and vegetables it would be a good idea to limit your consumption of red meat and saturated fats found in butter, peanuts and pork, exercise regularly and maintain your optimal weight.

THE SPECIAL NUTRIENTS AND REGULAR SCREENING

As they do with the prevention of breast and prostate cancer soy, lycopene, selenium, fish oil, green tea and resveratrol all have a role to play in the prevention of CRC. Another beneficial nutrient is lutein found in broccoli and dark-green vegetables such as spinach and lettuce, which has been shown to prevent the recurrence of CRC. Animal studies have shown that whey protein, lactoferrin, which is derived from whey, and pomegranate seed oil are also protective while two large human trials have demonstrated that 700mg a day of supplementary calcium reduces the risk of CRC. (130) (131) (132) (133) Yogurt, which has long been heralded as a health promoting agent, has shown some promise in animal studies as an anti-cancer agent with further evidence indicatin that beneficial bacteria such as lactobacillus rhamnosus GG, lactobacillus acidophilus, lactobacillus, casei, bifidobacterium lactis combined with sugars such as inulin and fructooligosaccharides have inhibitory effects on the growth of CRC.

Anti-inflammatory agents such as aspirin, non-steroidal anti-inflammatory medications and cox-2 inhibitors such as celecoxib have all been shown to reduce CRC, however, these can generate side-effects such as gastrointestinal bleeding, which would make natural agents such as curcumin and ginger more attractive.

While there is a consensus that regular screening via colonoscopy from the age of 40 is a good idea for those with first-degree relatives who have developed CRC there is still some debate concerning the type of screening procedures that all of us should undergo. If you're willing to subject yourself to the indignity of submitting a stool specimen this can be examined for the presence of bleeding from the bowel which would need further investigating by means of sigmoidoscopy or colonoscopy if this test is positive. Then there is the recently introduced virtual colonoscopy, which is a useful non-invasive way to identify any tumours of reasonable size via CT technology. A meeting of the Israeli gastroenterology society held in 2003 has championed the proposal that this sort of screening should commence from the age of 50. An annual stool test plus a 5-yearly sigmoidoscopy or colonoscopy would probably be the way to go. Whether this is embraced by the world medical community only time will tell.

Have a regular scope

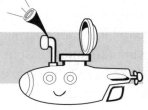

Preventing colorectal cancer

- Oestrogen
- Dehydroepiandrosterone (DHEA)
- Vitamin C 1 gram daily
- Vitamin D 1000i.u. daily
- Vitamin E consisting of mixed tocopherols 200- 400mg daily
- Vitamin E consisting of mixed tocotrienols 50mg daily
- Folic acid 400micrograms daily
- Beta-carotene 20mg daily
- Soybean products including miso, tofu and natto
- Cruciferous vegetables such as broccoli, Brussels sprouts, cabbage and cauliflower
- Lycopene 10-20mg daily
- Selenium 200micrograms daily
- Fish oils containing 120-360mg of EPA and 80-240mg of DHA daily
- Green tea 2- 4 cups daily
- Resveratrol 5-20mg daily
- Calcium 700mg daily
- Lutein 6mg daily
- Lactoferrin 250mg daily
- Whey protein 5 grams daily
- Pomegranate seed oil
- Yoghurt
- Lactobacillus rhamnosus GG, lactobacillus acidophilus, lactobacillus casei and bifidobacterium lactis combined with sugars such as inulin and fructooligosaccharides

TREATING COLORECTAL CANCER
HORMONES, VITAMINS, ANTIOXIDANTS, SPECIAL NUTRIENTS AND DIET

Melatonin, vitamin B6, vitamin D, vitamin E, lycopene, retinoic acid, quercetin, resveratrol, fish oil, green tea, calcium, calcium D-glucarate, curcumin, coriolus versicolor and modified citrus pectin all have their part to play in the treatment of CRC. These have been described in the preceding sections. Unfortunately most of the evidence for this is from animal and cell culture studies nevertheless the potential of these substances should not be underestimated. The same dietary principles that apply to the other cancers should be observed here. It's all about consuming vegetables, especially the green variety, low glycaemic fruits in moderation, the small fish, nuts, seeds and plenty of filtered water while limiting red meat, eggs and dairy. Regular exercise and maintaining your best weight would be ideal.

Treating colorectal cancer

- Melatonin 5-20mg daily
- Vitamin B6 200mg daily
- Vitamin D 3000-5000 i.u.daily
- Vitamin E mixed tocopherols 200-400mg daily
- Vitamin E mixed tocotrienols 50mg daily
- Lycopene 5-20mg daily
- Resveratrol 5-20mg daily
- Quercetin 500-1000mg daily

- Green tea 6 cups or 250-500mg daily
- Curcumin 200-400mg one to three times daily
- Modified citrus Pectin 20-30grams daily
- Retinoic acid 20mg daily
- Calcium 700-1000mg daily
- Calcium D-glucarate 400-1200mg daily
- Fish oil 2 grams daily
- Coriolus versicolor 3 grams daily

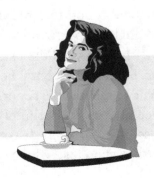

Green Tea is
Good for You

Here's a question. What do Sheila Jones aged 49 and ex-president Bill Clinton have in common? If you're guessing serious heart disease you'd be absolutely right. Sheila came to see me complaining of chest pain during her daily walk. Initially she didn't pay much attention to these uncomfortable feelings thinking that this was merely heartburn and that she shouldn't eat so much before her regular exercise routine. When the discomfort intensified she started to become a little worried and that's when I saw her. She had stopped her cholesterol-lowering medication as she thought it was making her rather tired.

Although her mother had died of a heart attack when she was just 59 Sheila never thought that this would happen to her. After all her life was going along pretty nicely. There were no financial worries. Her relationship with her husband was reasonably comfortable and she had taken very well to her new weight loss programme.

I performed the usual screening tests to make sure that she hadn't suffered a heart attack and when all was clear decided that the best course of action was for her to see a heart specialist as she definitely needed more testing to rule out the possibility of heart disease. Both her exercise EKG and the cardiac echo test, which scanned her heart, suggested that she had significant heart disease and just like it was for Bill Clinton the next step for her was to have an angiogram. This investigation provides an image of the blood vessels of the heart and while the ex-president had more than 90% blockage in all the major vessels providing blood to his heart only one of Sheila's was substantially clogged up. Sheila was lucky. Unlike Bill Clinton she didn't have to undergo a gruelling four-hour bypass operation. All she needed was the insertion of a new tube called a stent into the blood vessel that was occluded so that the blood supply to her heart muscle could be maintained. As is the routine she was then placed on aspirin and another statin medication to lower her cholesterol and she has also commenced a vitamin and antioxidant programme to minimise her chances of ever getting blocked arteries again.

Although Sheila's case is a touch unusual as she was rather young when she started to run into trouble, women do suffer from heart disease. This experience might start a little later in life but as women get older they start to catch up with men and with the current epidemic of obesity spreading throughout the western world there is every sign that women will soon be highly competitive with men with regard to heart attack statistics. As it now stands heart disease is the number one killer of both men and women. In the USA in 1999 there was one death from cardiovascular disease every 33 seconds.

Do you remember Jim, the patient I mentioned in the first chapter, who was suffering from what sounded like innocuous chest pain, was coerced into seeing me by his wife and 24 hours later he was dead? 50% of the time this is exactly what happens. Without any prior warning signs your first heart attack can be your last. In many ways Sheila and Bill Clinton were flirting with the angel of death. Both had a strong family history of heart disease, they shared a high cholesterol problem but didn't pay that much attention and each one of them thought that their chest pain was indigestion which would eventually go away. Quite fortuitously each consulted with their doctor before it was too late otherwise they might have become a heart attack victim and a fatal one at that as tragically did Jim.

You might not know this but atherosclerosis, which is as big a mouthful as it is the blockage of your blood vessels, starts as far back as the first decade of your life and intensifies as you get older. What you can do is reduce and even reverse these nasty blockages so that they cause you no harm. The truth is we probably know more about the events that lead to atherosclerosis and heart disease than we do most other disorders. We know the risk factors, we know how to measure them and we know how to deal with them.

The trouble is that most, like Sheila and Bill Clinton, don't pay much attention until those disturbing symptoms start to surface and even then they tend to be ignored. For a large proportion of us this can be a tragic error. The way to prevent this from happening is so simple. Once you understand what places you at risk you can then undergo the relevant investigations to see whether you have any of these risk factors and you can then take the necessary steps to minimise your risk. You will discover how hormones and vitamins have a considerable impact on the outcome of heart disease.

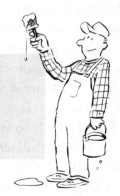

You'd better look after the wall of your blood vessels

RISK FACTORS FOR ATHEROSCLEROSIS

Here there are two major factors that you have to address. The first is referred to as endothelial dysfunction and the second is far more lethal and is termed plaque rupture. Everyone knows about the dangers of high cholesterol and elevated blood pressure. Most patients when they consult with me want to be reassured that these are within the normal range. But this is only a small part of the story. Half of the time you can have a heart attack with a totally normal cholesterol reading.

What you really have to know about is how the endothelium, which is the lining of your blood vessels becomes damaged and how the plaque or the ball of fat that accumulates inside those vessels as a result of this disruption becomes vulnerable to rupture. Each and every one of us has some plaque build-up. We all have fat or plaque, which is accumulating inside the lining of our blood vessels on an ongoing basis. Obviously we don't want excessive aggregation of this substance as our blood vessels will then become progressively obstructed which can limit the blood supply to the chambers of our heart.

However it is the vulnerable plaque or the plaque which is prone to rupture that can be even more lethal. Plaque rupture leads to the massing of a vast number of cells which can totally block the blood vessels serving your heart muscle leading to a massive heart attack. In 50% of cases this can be the first and only indication that you have some form of heart disease and tragically you might not have an opportunity to take any evasive action. It is this kind of blockage, which occurs without warning, that can be deadly. However if you want to know where it all starts it is endothelial dysfunction or damage to the lining of your blood vessels that is the primary instigator of heart disease. Endothelial dysfunction is the earliest event that gets atherosclerosis and the build-up of plaque going. What is it exactly that causes endothelial dysfunction?

THE DIET

We all know that eating too much fat is bad for our cholesterol levels. What fat also does is wreak havoc with your endothelium and the more fat you consume the worse this state of affairs becomes. On any given day the average American would consume between 20-70grams of fat with each meal, which is a whopping amount of this lethal substance. If you have a liking for fast-food items such as muffins, Danish pastries, doughnuts, fried chicken and hamburgers, followed by high-fat ice creams or you live on red meat and dairy products then your levels of fats will rise quite precipitously.

In the USA trans fatty acids (TFAs) found in margarines will exacerbate this problem whereas in Australia TFAs were eliminated from margarines after 1996 and no longer pose a threat. The notion that fats can be so potentially toxic would constitute a serious setback for the advocates of the high protein, high fat, low carbohydrate diet. Even though this type of diet might help with weight loss having your endothelium constantly bathed in oceans of fat can erode the lining of your blood vessels, which can be extremely dangerous.

There's a range of other reasons for the difficulties that you might have in processing fat. Eating lots of fat becomes even more detrimental as you get older, or if you're obese, are a post-menopausal woman, have a family history of heart disease, have had a previous heart attack, spend most of your time on the computer or watching television and have a passion for refined carbohydrates such as sweets, chocolate, cake and biscuits. If you really want to limit the unfavourable effects of fats then you need to restrict your consumption of this substance to not more than 20grams per meal which really isn't that difficult if you set your mind to it.

While you're restricting your cholesterol-rich foods found in dairy products and red meat you also want to go easy on the egg consumption. Eggs can increase high-density lipoprotein (HDL) which is the good cholesterol but unfortunately they also tend to raise total cholesterol and low-density lipoprotein (LDL), the bad cholesterol, by even greater amounts which offsets all the benefits as far as your heart is concerned. (1) This is especially true for women who for some reason seem to suffer more from the adverse effects of excessive egg consumption. (2) If you want to play it safe then don't have more than four-five eggs per week and if you really want to cut down on your enjoyment of this food then eliminate the yolk, which is the source of cholesterol.

Just to follow up on the problem with sugar, if you have difficulty metabolising this substance this can pose tangible problems for your heart. The way to check this is with a fasting 2-hour glucose tolerance test, which also measures insulin. I've mentioned this before in the weight loss chapter. Normally your fasting glucose would be around 4-5 mmol/L, which would go up to 7mmol/L one hour after a glucose drink and this would then come back down to around 5mmol/L at the 2 hour mark. If your scores are above this range particularly after one or two hours then you are suffering from what is called post-prandial hyperglyceamia or high blood sugar which leads to the increased production of free radicals and these then have a glorious time disrupting your endothelium. Ensuring that your glucose metabolism is within range is mightily important for your heart.

CHOLESTEROL, LOW DENSITY LIPOPROTEIN (LDL), HIGH DENSITY LIPOPROTEIN (HDL), TRIGLYCERIDES AND APOPROTEINS A-1 AND B

We all know that having too much cholesterol in the diet is bad but it's really the LDL cholesterol that does all the damage to your endothelium. Ideally you want to maintain your LDL cholesterol below 130mg/dL, which is around 3mmol/L, but the experts in the USA are going one step further. If you have added risk factors which make you even more vulnerable including cigarette smoking, high blood pressure, an HDL<40mg/dL or <1mmol/L, a family history of early heart disease (<55 in male first-degree relative; <65 in female first-degree relative) or you're a male older than 45 or a female older than 55 then you need to aim for an even lower LDL below 100mg/dL or 2.5mmol/L. (3)

It's not just LDL that you have to guard against. There are also different types of LDLs and some are more harmful than others. The bad guys are small, dense LDL, oxidised LDL and very low-density lipoprotein (VLDL). Large, buoyant LDL is thought to be much less harmful. In fact it is the small, dense variety that is much more susceptible to oxidation or attack by free radicals and it is this form of oxidised LDL that causes ongoing damage to the endothelium. In Australia, laboratories don't measure small, dense LDL yet, which is a pity, but if you are overweight and especially if you suffer from the metabolic syndrome or syndrome X which is associated with insulin resistance and you have high triglycerides and low HDL chances are you have a high proportion of small, dense LDL which is rapidly becoming oxidised.

Oxidised LDL also increases with exposure to saturated fats found in meat and dairy, deep-fried foods, packaged biscuits, cakes and pastries, heavy metals such as mercury, lead, arsenic and cadmium, excessive iron and copper exposure and even emotional stress. Negative emotions have a substantial impact on the health of your endothelium. Depression, grief, anxiety, isolation, hostility and excessive expression of anger which would manifest in ongoing road rage or extreme irritability at waiting in line all unite to increase your risk for developing heart disease. Resentment and concealed anger are also highly detrimental. American psychoneuroimmunoendocrinology (this is the longest word in this book and easier to say after two glasses of bourbon) expert Dr Robert A. Anderson advises that anger be expressed in a socially acceptable way such as pounding a cushion, or beating a mattress with a bat or by acknowledging the emotion and then letting it go without imparting excessive blame. Anger can often result from needs that are frustrated, which suggests that identifying the need and vocalising it might make you feel less angry. Forgiveness is another method to deal with unresolved anger.

Still Dr Anderson suggests that in the interest of our hearts we all aim to become "certified adults" which is someone who has "fully accepted him/herself; has resolved stressful past issues; maintains a centred emotional posture; and balances concern for him/herself with that for others." That person is more likely to be developing his/her full potential and may also be said to be " fully alive." Just in case you don't know such a person it's OK. As long as you are heading in this direction you're on the right path.

While you're busy organising your emotional balance and you want to find out whether your blood stream is saturated with oxidised LDL there is a blood test performed by American laboratories such as Immunosciences located at the website www.immunoscienceslab.com which measures antibodies to oxidised LDL. These go up when there are elevated levels of oxidised LDL in your body and are said to be associated with progression of atherosclerosis.

High VLDL also harbours cholesterol-rich particles, which it passes on to LDL. To find out whether you are troubled by high levels of VLDL you need to have your apoprotein B (apoB) levels measured. This is a protein which transports LDL and VLDL around the body. Each VLDL and LDL particle contains one molecule of apoB and therefore your total plasma apoB count would add up to all the particles that can do you harm. In other words, apart from your LDL and triglyceride levels, assessing your apoB status will provide you with added information about your risk. Levels greater than 130mg/dL or 3 mmol/L would place you in the danger zone. While apoB would be B for bad apoA-1 stands for apple (an easy way to remember this) indicating goodness. ApoA-1 works in tandem with HDL and helps this molecule to remove the bad cholesterol from the lining of your blood vessels. Maintaining healthy levels of apoA-1 and reducing the harmful apoB is critically important.

Triglycerides are another form of fat, which have the ability to do some harm when present in excessive amounts. When fat is absorbed and deposited in the liver triglycerides are extracted, which then become a transport medium for cholesterol around your body. Elevated serum triglyceride levels are associated with small, dense LDL and low HDL levels. Once your triglycerides go up LDL becomes even more dangerous and HDL less protective. This often happens in the context of metabolic syndrome or obesity. A high triglyceride level would be >150mg/dL or >1.7mmol/L.

Australian cardiologist Dr Ross Walker, who also has an interest in natural therapies, indicates in his book 'The Cell Factor' that elevated triglycerides are commonly found in overweight people, those with liver disease especially the alcoholic variety, diabetics and those with an underactive thyroid gland.

HDL
is the good guy

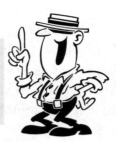

Most would know that HDL is the good guy in this story with the power to unblock your blood vessels and remove all the nasty cholesterol from the danger spots to your liver where it can be harmlessly eliminated. HDL also prevents the oxidation of LDL and is involved in a whole range of beneficial behaviours, which essentially prevent plaque from growing or rupturing. It has been estimated that every 1mg/dL or 0.3mmol/L increase in HDL reduces heart disease risk by 3%. (4)

One of the most powerful ways to raise your HDL levels is via a B vitamin called niacin. To give you some idea of the comparison, statins, the cholesterol-lowering medications, increase HDL by 5-12% while niacin does the job by approximately 15-30%. Policosanol made from sugar cane extract is another natural substance with the ability to increase HDL. Regular exercise and weight loss will also boost HDL. HDL starts to become protective when your levels exceed 60mg/dL or 1.5mmol/L.

In case you think I've forgotten about cholesterol this substance also has a hefty influence on the growth of plaque. 30% of your body's cholesterol comes from your diet, while the other 70% depends on the functioning of your liver, your genetic inheritance and the efficiency of your bowel's eliminating powers. Your liver manufactures cholesterol but is also, along with your bowel, responsible for dispensing with this compound once your body no longer has any use for it. It is for this reason that it is so important to have a fully operational liver and a bowel that works regularly. This is why a herb such as globe artichoke, which improves liver function, also reduces cholesterol levels.

Once your cholesterol exceeds 280mg/dL or 6.5mmol/L it is highly likely that hereditary factors are coming in to play especially if your mother or father suffered a heart attack before the age of 60. In this scenario your doctor will be inclined to place you on cholesterol-lowering medications like the statin drugs, which have their limitations and are not without side-effects.

A good friend of mine who has just turned 51 and has a strong family history of heart disease started taking a statin three years ago when he returned a cholesterol reading of 7.1. I don't think he did much in the way of vitamin supplementation and he didn't pay much attention to his hormonal levels either. A few months before I wrote this segment he noticed that he was becoming increasingly breathless when walking his dogs. He didn't think much of this as he had rather energetic animals and it was only when he began to develop crushing chest pain that he realised he was in strife. One cardiac echo and angiogram later and he found himself facing the same quadruple bypass operation that Bill Clinton had to negotiate. Sometimes medication will get you out of trouble but if you are going to rely on pharmaceuticals alone to protect you then you may be headed for trouble. You may need a much more holistic approach than that.

LIPOPROTEIN (a)

Closely aligned with LDL in the axis of evil to increase your risk of developing atherosclerosis is lipoprotein (a). Lipoprotein (a) is formed by joining a fat that is very similar in structure to LDL to a protein called apolipoprotein (a) together with apo (B) which you already know is one of the bad guys. Once your lipoprotein (a) exceeds 33mg/dL (0.11mmol/L) and you also have a raised LDL then your risk of developing coronary artery disease increases. (5)

The trouble is that the tendency to develop raised lipoprotein (a) is inherited for the most part and is also extremely difficult to reduce. Some experts claim that a deficiency of vitamin C and the amino acid lysine will exacerbate this problem. Supplementing with vitamin C and lysine together with omega-3 fatty acids might have a positive effect while testosterone in men and oestrogen in women can also reduce lipoprotein (a). High doses of the B vitamin niacin (2 grams per day or more) can decrease blood levels of lipoprotein (a) by 20-30%. If you're taking DHEA you need to have your lipoprotein (a) levels monitored as there is one study indicating that supplementing with this hormone can increase lipoprotein (a) in men and the same might happen in women. (6)

HOMOCYSTEINE

Homocysteine is an amino acid, which is a type of protein that is derived from another amino acid called methionine, found mostly in animal protein, and is usually pretty innocuous. In the normal course of events homocysteine is converted back to methionine or makes another amino acid, which goes by the name of cysteine. For these interconversions to proceed without hitch vitamins B6, B12 and folic acid are needed. However, if these vitamins are lacking, homocysteine levels start to escalate and it is raised homocysteine that can tamper with your endothelium, increase dangerous oxidised LDL and activate all the other factors that lead to the accumulation of plaque and the progression of atherosclerosis.

Aside from vitamin deficiencies there are other factors that increase homocysteine levels including being a male or a postmenopausal woman, advancing age, excessive consumption of alcohol and coffee, low thyroid function, lack of exercise, obesity and a genetic mutation of the enzyme methylene tetrahydrofolate reductase which is responsible for making folic acid function effectively and is present in 10-20% of Caucasians. One study has even shown that those who have this gene have a 21% increased risk of developing heart disease. (7) Homocysteine should be maintained at a level which is less than 10umoles/L and the closer this value is to the lower end of the range, which is 5umoles/L, the safer you will be.

Vitamins B6, B12, folic acid, a substance called betaine or trimethylglycine, which was first discovered in the juice of sugar beets, and oestrogen used in hormone replacement therapy have the power to lower homocysteine. If you have tried the vitamin and folic acid strategy and your homocysteine level has not decreased then you may be suffering from the methylene tetrahydrofolate reductase gene problem and you would need to utilise betaine, which reduces homocysteine via an alternative biochemical pathway.

INFLAMMATION

If there's one factor that you need to be extremely wary of it's inflammation. This is the incendiary process that initiates endothelial dysfunction, promotes the accumulation of plaque and finally leads to plaque rupture. Inflammation is the unifying force that gives expression to all those factors that stimulate the development of heart disease. Oxidised LDL, elevated cholesterol levels, raised blood pressure, high blood sugar, obesity and infections operate primarily by increasing inflammation. Even fat cells harbour inflammatory molecules, which find their way to the lining of your blood vessels where they instigate atherosclerosis. Bacteria such as Chlamydia pneumoniae, which comes from your lungs, and helicobacter pylori found in your stomach both common sources of infection that lead to inflammation, have been located in atheroscerotic plaque.

If you're not fastidious about brushing your teeth and regular flossing you might have to improve your dental hygiene, as there's a study which connects poor oral health with coronary heart disease. (8) There are those who postulate that fungi might be an underlying cause of heart disease and there is also a possibility that the ubiquitous candida albicans might be implicated. (9) Once inflammation gets going it develops a momentum that can single-handedly propel you towards a cardiovascular catastrophe. You don't even have to have high cholesterol or severely blocked arteries to be in danger. Once inflammation sets in your risk of having a heart attack increases quite dramatically.

If you want to know whether inflammation is establishing itself in your blood vessels, and I'm clearly suggesting that it's in your best interests to have this knowledge so that you can take the necessary steps to cut short this process, then all you need is a simple blood test. Highly sensitive C-reactive protein (HS-CRP) is a substance that is produced predominantly in your liver and is a reliable marker of inflammation. Even if your LDL and cholesterol levels are normal once your HS-CRP levels are elevated your risk increases. An HS-CRP level less than 1mg/L indicates a low risk, 1-3 a moderate risk and a reading greater than 3.0mg/L a high risk. (10) For some reason an elevated HS-CRP has more serious ramifications for women and there's a study which has revealed that when comparing this risk factor with the other important predisposing factors such as high cholesterol and raised blood pressure HS-CRP was the strongest predictor of risk for cardiovascular events in women, which indicates that it's critically important that if you're a women you need to have your HS-CRP measured. (11)

If you want to obtain a comprehensive inflammatory profile, there are other inflammatory markers that can be quantified including interleukin-6, fibrinogen and the ratio of arachidonic acid, which is a fat derived mostly from meat and is thought to be pro-inflammatory, to eicosapentaenoic acid which comes from fish and is anti-inflammatory. You might find that your HS-CRP is only modestly elevated and including these other indicators will give you added information about your inflammatory status. These are not investigations that are commonly instituted by your doctor, however if you want to give yourself every chance of preventing heart disease these are certainly steps you need to consider.

Naturally it's not a good idea to determine the HS-CRP or the other inflammatory indices in isolation. You would need to have all the factors evaluated that contribute to heart disease such as LDL, homocysteine, insulin resistance etc to get a complete picture of the interventions that you need to introduce to minimise your risk and lower your HS-CRP if your levels are high. As a general rule though there are studies which show that a Mediterranean diet comprising lots of fruit and vegetables especially onions, garlic and red grapes together with a weight loss programme, regular exercise and smoking cessation will reduce HS-CRP levels. Adding the regular consumption of anti-inflammatory herbs such as ginger and turmeric won't go astray either.

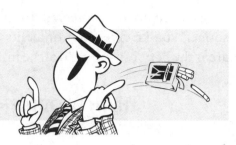

Observe non smoking areas

CIGARETTE SMOKING

Everyone knows that cigarette smoking causes lung cancer, which makes it rather difficult to comprehend why this deadly habit is so widespread. What most might not realise is that smoking increases the risk of a heart attack. Although this is disturbing information it would suffice if this matter ended there. After all there is a warning on each pack of cigarettes that this practice is bad for your health. Unfortunately the toxic fumes emanating from cigarette smoke have the potential to harm all of us. Passive smoking or the environmental exposure to tobacco smoke has been shown to damage the lining of blood vessels, compromise blood flow to the chambers of the heart, stiffen the aorta, the major vessel that supplies the body with blood, compromise the heart rate, decrease antioxidant capacity and make blood thicker and stickier. For those continually exposed to cigarette smoke in the home, the workplace or recreational facilities the likelihood of having a heart attack doubles.

Does this upset you? It should. It's extremely heartening (if you'll excuse the pun) to see that local councils in Sydney are taking it upon themselves to prohibit smoking not only indoors but also in the outside area of restaurants. In the USA the city of Helena instituted a public smoking ban in 2002 and found that hospital admissions as a result of heart attacks were reduced by almost half. The message is plain and simple. All of us need to be protected from cigarette smoke and the sooner smoke-free environments are introduced in public areas the better shape we'll all be in.

HIGH BLOOD PRESSURE

We used to be rather liberal with what we regarded as high blood pressure with readings of 140/90 mm Hg and above being considered abnormal. Now experts consider a much lower value to be the cut-off point. In fact in 2003 in the USA the Seventh Report of the Joint National Committee on the Prevention, Detection, Evaluation and treatment of High Blood Pressure suggested that the risk of cardiovascular disease actually begins at 115/75 mm Hg and doubles with each increment of 20/10 mm Hg. A consistently elevated blood pressure is detrimental to the lining of your blood vessels and increases your risk for heart attack and stroke. I have found in my practice that going the natural route for lowering blood pressure is not always 100% effective but certainly worth a try. Weight loss, consuming more than five serves of fruit and vegetables daily, limiting your intake of animal products and processed foods that are high in salt, regular exercise and meditation and supplementing with a team of nutrients including vitamins C and E, magnesium, calcium, omega-3 fatty acids found in either fish oil or ground flaxseeds, the amino acids L-arginine and taurine, coenzyme Q10 and the herbs garlic and hawthorn is an approach that might work for you. If this cocktail seems a little complex you're welcome to try the ACE inhibitor medications, which also have anti-inflammatory and antioxidant properties and are thought to have anti-ageing potential.

DIABETES AND THE METABOLIC SYNDROME

If you are overweight and your blood pressure is raised it is highly likely that your are also suffering from the metabolic syndrome or syndrome X. This condition is associated with insulin resistance, the aggregation of small, dense LDL cholesterol particles, elevated triglycerides and a number of other proinflammatory factors, which significantly increase your risk for developing heart disease. In the USA almost ¼ of the adult population suffer from the metabolic syndrome which amounts to the colossal figure of 48,000,000 people. In the western world obesity is becoming a burgeoning problem with massive ramifications for health care delivery worldwide.

Diabetics are prone to having elevated triglyceride levels and excess sugar attaches itself to LDL making this substance more damaging to the endothelium.

INCREASED CLOTTING FACTORS

When you cut yourself, platelets and other molecules in your bloodstream known as clotting factors help your blood to congeal which prevents you from bleeding endlessly. These same factors can congregate around the areas where plaque is accumulating and they also have a tendency to make your blood sludgier which makes you more susceptible to developing blocked arteries. There are a number of these factors including fibrinogen, activated factor V11, plasminogen activator inhibitor-1, factor V Leiden and others which aren't routinely evaluated but do need to be investigated if you suffer from recurrent blood clots.

Risk factors for heart disease

- Excessive consumption of saturated fats, trans fatty acids, refined carbohydrates and eggs
- Free radical excess
- High cholesterol, LDL especially oxidised and small, dense LDL, apoprotein B and triglycerides
- Low HDL
- Ongoing depression, grief, anxiety, isolation, hostility and unabated anger
- Raised lipoprotein (a)
- Elevated homocysteine
- Family history of heart disease
- Inflammation
- Raised HS-CRP
- Cigarette smoking and passive exposure to tobacco smoke
- High blood pressure
- Diabetes
- Insulin resistance
- An increase in clotting factors

Once you've covered all these bases, and you can identify most of the factors that lead to heart disease with simple blood tests, it is also highly beneficial to discover whether you have vulnerable plaque.   This is the kind of plaque that is most dangerous.   Once plaque ruptures then a host of molecules and clotting factors swarm to this area, which results in a critical obstruction of blood flow. This can lead to a major heart attack and tragically in some cases even sudden death. Here's a case in point.

Many years ago when I was studying at university there was a fellow student I fancied but being the shy, retiring type I didn't make my feelings known to her. After we graduated we went our separate ways and through the grapevine I heard that she had married and had immigrated to Australia. It was purely a matter of coincidence that I followed in her footsteps and I often wondered when I would bump into her. After not seeing her for 30 years I attended a movie premier a few months ago and there she was looking not much different from the same attractive young lady I had courted in my mind all those years back. Needless to say I went up to her and introduced myself and with much excitement we soon found ourselves chatting away and reminiscing about times gone by. As you would I asked her how married life was treating her thinking that she had settled into connubial bliss and was living happily ever after. In a rather matter of fact fashion which made it even the more awkward for me she announced that her husband had died quite suddenly some years ago. Apparently he had gone on his daily jog, without any prior warning developed chest pain and by the time his running partner alerted the paramedics it was too late. You can imagine that the conversation became a little uncomfortable after that startling revelation and having exchanged further bumbling pleasantries we swapped phone numbers and drifted back into the anonymity of the evening.

If you're wondering whether this story has a romantic ending I haven't contacted her since that night but the real point I'm making is that this awful tragedy might have been averted had her husband undergone the necessary tests to see whether he was at risk. There are a number of factors that make your plaque more vulnerable.

These include:
• The accumulation of cholesterol
• The deposition of small, dense and oxidised LDL together with lipoprotein (a) within the plaque
• Increasing inflammation
• The build-up of free radicals
• Emotional stress
• High blood pressure

These are the factors which you have to minimise if you want to eliminate the possibility of sustaining plaque rupture and keeling over while going for your daily constitutional, (your walk or your run). However if you want to go the full Monty and discover whether you are sitting on a time bomb with plaque just waiting to detonate then it just so happens that there are investigations, which will provide you with that kind of information.

A CAROTID ULTRASOUND

A simple scan of the arteries in your neck can provide you with vital information about the build-up of plaque in these vessels, which correlates quite substantially with the type of plaque you have in the major vessels that supply your heart. In the hands of a skilled ultrasonographer this investigation can also be used to estimate vulnerable plaque that has a chance of rupturing. Surprisingly not many doctors employ this method to help establish whether their patients are at risk.

CORONARY CT SCAN

A special type of CT scan called the electron beam CT can be used to quantify the amount of calcium that you have in your coronary arteries which has been found to predict whether you are at risk of having a heart attack. High calcium scores indicate the presence of extensive plaque, some of which will be vulnerable and will unquestionably place you in the danger zone. There is even evidence that coronary artery calcification is a more powerful predictor of cardiovascular events than all the risk factors mentioned earlier. (12) Another more sophisticated type of CT scan called the multidetector low spiral CT scan also has the potential to specifically identify vulnerable plaque.

MAGNETIC RESONANCE IMAGING (MRI)

Although this has not been introduced yet, high-resolution MRI is the new technology that will provide very clear pictures of plaque that is at high risk of disruption. This will allow your doctor to intervene much more aggressively to ward off any impending disaster.

Rather than rely on any singular investigation my suggestion is to have all the tests I mentioned in the risk factor section and then proceed to an ultrasound of your carotids and a CT scan of your coronary arteries.

This is exactly the course of events that Patricia, a 45 year-old teacher with a strong family history of heart disease, followed. Her total cholesterol level was 6.2 and her LDL 4.2, both of which were elevated. Her homocysteine reading was 10.5, which was within the normal range, which is 10-15 but could do with some lowering. Her lipopotein (a) score was normal. She did not have insulin resistance but her HS-CRP was 2, which placed her in the moderate risk zone indicating that some inflammation was present. She did not have the blood test which assesses antibodies to oxidised LDL although this would have been useful, as this test is not yet done in Australia and would have needed the services of an American laboratory. Her carotid ultrasound indicated that she had some presence of plaque. This was further confirmed by her coronary CT scan, which indicated that her calcium score placed her in the high-risk category for succumbing to a heart attack

Her cardiologist was insistent that she go on aspirin and a statin medication to lower her cholesterol and minimise her chances of having any critical cardiovascular event. Patricia wasn't too keen on jumping into any pharmaceutical approach and was wary of the potential side-effects of these medications so she opted for a more natural approach. She changed her diet by reducing her consumption of red meat and started to have more fish. She had been promising to commence an exercise programme but had struggled with finding the motivation. Once she received the results of all her tests it didn't take much for her to agree that regular exercise was a good idea. To lower her cholesterol and LDL she started taking policosanol, to which she added vitamins C and E to neutralise any possible accumulation of free radicals. To address her less than optimal homocysteine level, a B vitamin complex including folic acid was instituted, and to combat the existence of inflammation we introduced a herbal compound including ginger and turmeric.

When she returned after 3 months of adhering to this programme it was rather gratifying to see her cholesterol come down to 5.4 and her LDL to 3.5. Her homocysteine had decreased slightly to 8.9 and her HS-CRP, while still in the moderate risk zone had moderately improved at 1.5. With these positive trends she was encouraged to remain on her programme and her risk factors have continued to lessen which has provided her with even more motivation to continue.

Once you've had all your tests you can then adopt a strategy to minimise your risk factors, reduce the plaque that you've accumulated and most importantly prevent the plaque that's already there from becoming vulnerable to rupture. Here are the natural means that you can adopt to achieve these goals.

THE HORMONES
OESTROGEN

Most women don't know this but heart disease not breast cancer is the leading cause of death for the female population of the western world. Before the menopausal transition the incidence of heart disease for women is much lower than that of their male counterparts but by the time women reach the age of 65 the risk of succumbing to a heart attack accelerates so dramatically that women have practically caught up to men. We think that this might have a lot to do with all the benefits of oestrogen which are missed after menopause once the body produces much less of this hormone. Oestrogen has a wide range of positive effects on the cardiovascular system including the reduction of LDL, neutralising free radicals which limits the accumulation of oxidised LDL, inhibiting plaque build-up, reducing homocysteine, lipoprotein (a) and cholesterol, lowering blood pressure, increasing HDL and protecting the endothelium. (13) (14)

If the Women's Health Initiative study which demonstrated an increased risk of heart attack in those women who took Premarin, the oestrogen derived from horse's urine, and Provera doesn't really support the notion that oestrogen is protective, it probably has a lot to do with the fact that the wrong form of hormones was used when it was already too late. Another study, which incorporated oestrogen in the form of oestradiol, showed that when this hormone was administered soon after menopause the progression of atherosclerosis was prevented. (15)

This is the core point. Using oestrogen either in the form of oestradiol or oestriol, the weaker oestrogen, soon after menopause before heart disease has a chance to set in might be the ideal way to nip this whole process in the bud. You might realise by now that I'm an advocate of hormone replacement and, as you would expect, experts around the world are reluctant to support the use of hormones for the long-term prevention of heart disease citing the use of other means for doing this such as the statin medications where appropriate. I have patients who have been taking hormones for over 20 years ever since they went through menopause and they are doing very well. The dose of hormones that I use is 1-2mg of Triest which is the combination of oestradiol, oestrone and oestriol in the form of a troche or a cream, ½ of which is taken in the morning followed by the other half in the late afternoon. For those women who need a stronger dose of oestradiol I use 1mg of oestradiol on its own either in the form of a troche or the cream.

PROGESTERONE

Natural progesterone and not the progestogen found in Provera which is thought to be detrimental to the female heart, is another hormone that might do a lot of good with regard to preventing heart disease. Rather than get in the way of oestrogen, which Provera appears to do, natural progesterone actually assists oestrogen's beneficial effects on plaque reduction, improves blood supply and preserves the favourable effects that oestrogen has on HDL. The amount of progesterone that I prescribe is either 200-400mg of this hormone in the form of a troche or 20-40mg in the form of a cream.

TESTOSTERONE

Cardiovascular disease by a long margin is the highest cause of death in men and generally affects the male sex at a younger age than women. If oestrogen gives women a protective edge could it be that testosterone does the exact opposite for men? Those who are favourably disposed towards testosterone, and I would count myself as one of those as it's difficult to fathom how a hormone which is so inextricably linked to male well-being could also have the gumption to bring about our demise, would look at all the studies and identify all the benefits that this hormone brings to the cardiovascular system. Advantages, some of which I've already mentioned in this book, include testosterone's ability to lower cholesterol, lipoprotein (a) and LDL, maintain HDL levels, stimulate weight loss, make it more difficult for blood to clot and reduce the accumulation of plaque. (16)

By a strange quirk of nature testosterone also has the power to encourage the early formation of plaque (which might explain the head start that men have on women) and to further balance the ledger testosterone's mischief-making include its propensity to lower HDL and stimulate blood clotting which has been demonstrated in some studies. (17) Testosterone can also lower and elevate blood pressure, limit inflammation and promote the activity of inflammatory cells. If you think we are dealing with a hormone that has schizophrenic tendencies you're not wrong. There's a lot we still don't understand about the workings of this complex hormone.

What this does appear to tell us is that heart disease in men might be initiated earlier in life when testosterone levels are high. There is even a suggestion that exposure to high levels of maternal testosterone in the womb might predispose to the development of atherosclerosis later in life. Athletes or body builders who take testosterone when their bodies are producing enough of this hormone might be flirting with danger if this is the case.

If your testosterone levels are low and you are going to increase this hormone then you need to keep a watchful eye on all those factors that fall under testosterone's sphere of influence including your cholesterol levels, inflammation and your blood's clotting potential. You also need to ensure that your testosterone levels remain within range and are not boosted to excess.

A healthy dose of testosterone would be 25-50mg a day in divided doses either via a cream or a troche.

GROWTH HORMONE

Growth hormone is not commonly viewed as a boon for the cardiovascular system. However, if your levels are really low, then supplementing with this hormone can make it easier for you to lose weight and increase your HDL levels while lowering cholesterol and LDL. In ageing laboratory animals growth hormone appears to make the heart pump more effectively and improve blood flow. (18) There is also a suggestion in some studies that the decline in growth hormone production with ageing might promote atherosclerosis. (19) If you are going to commence with growth hormone supplementation then a good initial dose would be ½-¾ of an international unit daily.

DEHYDROEPIANDROSTERONE (DHEA)

Like testosterone DHEA also has a dual personality with one study indicating that this hormone has the ability to lower cholesterol in 60 to 70 yr old women while others indicate that DHEA can reduce HDL and possibly increase lipoprotein (a). (20) (21) (22) There is also evidence that DHEA can initiate plaque formation in a fashion similar to that of testosterone suggesting that men need to be especially cautious when supplementing with this hormone especially when the body is adequately supplied with DHEA. (23) Taking DHEA would not appear to be a problem when levels are low.   If this is the case for men 25mg of DHEA daily would be a healthy dose while for women 10-25 mg would be adequate. Ensuring that DHEA does not lead to excessive oestrogen levels in men is also important and here taking aromatase inhibitors including such substances as flaxseed, resveratrol and quercetin would be prudent.

THYROID HORMONE

Inadequate production of thyroid hormone can also raise cholesterol levels and increase heart disease risk. Lipoprotein (a) and homocysteine go up when thyroid hormone levels are low. (24) (25) I've indicated in chapter two that it is essential to have a complete thyroid evaluation including TSH, T3, T4 and reverse T3 and to pay particular attention to symptoms such as cold hands and feet which suggest that your thyroid hormone levels are low.   There isn't one specific regimen for thyroid hormone replacement with the appropriate treatment depending largely on the resolution of your symptoms and the correction of your thyroid hormone levels.

Hormones are highly complex influential chemicals, which can benefit the cardiovascular system in many different ways but also have the potential to be harmful especially when boosted to excess. For women being overweight, having too much testosterone and too little oestrogen increase the risk of having a heart attack as demonstrated by a study carried out in Australia. (26) For men having a surplus of testosterone especially earlier in life might be counterproductive. This is why it is a good idea to have your hormones monitored while you are on hormone treatment to ensure that they remain within safe limits along with the tests which measure cholesterol, lipoprotein (a) and all the other factors that are modified by hormones.

THE VITAMINS
VITAMIN E

This vitamin has such enormous potential to prevent heart disease that the studies, which have delivered conflicting results, are somewhat disappointing. While there is good evidence that vitamin E can curtail the development of atherosclerosis and even stabilise vulnerable plaque, which is a highly desirable outcome, there is also testament to the limitations of vitamin E with some trials showing that together with vitamin C and beta-carotene this vitamin can make things worse. (27) (28) (29) (30) If you're in favour of vitamin supplementation like myself then there are all sorts of reasons that you can invoke to discredit the negative studies and support the positive ones.

What is clear is that vitamin E is a highly complex compound comprised of a number of different substances called tocopherols and tocotrienols found in nuts, seeds and oils, which we don't consume in large amounts. The clinical trials in which vitamin E performed poorly only used one part of this vitamin called alpha-tocopherol which is like fielding a basketball team with only one player and still anticipating victory.

Unless you're playing the young Michael Jordan against a team of midgets expecting a winning result would be highly presumptuous and yet this was exactly the kind of game that a number of esteemed scientists were playing. Gamma-tocopherol, a highly significant component of vitamin E, and the different tocotrienols of which there are four found predominantly in palm oil, have been shown to inhibit and more impressively reverse plaque formation and yet these were omitted from the negative trials.

To add insult to injury the American Heart Association in a policy statement has ignored all the beneficial evidence and has concluded that the existing scientific data does not support the use of vitamins or antioxidant supplements for the prevention and treatment of heart disease. They go on to claim that if you consume adequate amounts of fruits, vegetables, whole grains and nuts then you are going to be supplied with all the protective nutrients you need.

This is all very well if the produce you consume is fresh, organic and in-season and you have a perfect digestive process ready to absorb all those vital substances but for most of us this is simply not the case. Time and again in my practice I see those patients who are lacking in essential nutrients. The investigations they undergo confirm this. I believe that we all need supplementary vitamins and antioxidants and as far as the heart is concerned extra vitamin E would be one of the mainstays of this programme. 200g daily of a mixed tocopherol complex containing alpha, gamma and the other tocopherols together with 50mg of the four tocotrienols would be a good maintenance dose.

VITAMIN C

The point about vitamins is that they operate best when combined with other protective nutrients. This is especially true for vitamin C which functions optimally when working together with vitamin E as well as coenzyme Q10 and alpha-lipoic acid. The study, which showed that vitamin E can stabilize vulnerable plaque, also incorporated vitamin C illustrating the wisdom of using these two vitamins together to attack that menacing mound of fat that is preparing to block up your blood vessels. Vitamin C also prevents LDL from becoming oxidised and lowers cholesterol in some studies making this vitamin a worthwhile investment in its own right. A protective dose of vitamin C would be 1000-2000mg daily.

THE B VITAMINS

Vitamins B6, B12 and folic acid are needed to lower homocysteine but the B vitamin with the ability to do the most good by a country mile is niacin or vitamin B3. Niacin is the most potent agent for raising HDL while at the same time lowering LDL, converting harmful small dense LDL to large buoyant LDL which is far more benign, inhibiting the oxidation of LDL, lowering lipoprotein (a) and triglycerides and making blood flow more easily. Niacin improves endothelial function, reduces inflammation, increases plaque stability and makes it harder for blood to clot. If ever there were a vitamin which could sweep all the Oscars niacin would have to be the number one candidate. Unfortunately niacin is not without its downside as it does cause flushing at higher doses, which can be quite uncomfortable and this vitamin can have adverse effects on the liver and raise blood sugar levels.

One way to minimise these negatives is to take a lower dose of the sustained release form of niacin known as inositol hexanicotinate. I suggest starting off with 500mg twice daily and you can increase your dosage if your cholesterol levels do not improve. While you are doing this tracking your liver function and blood glucose levels would be advisable.

THE DIET AND EXERCISE

In addition to optimising your hormone profile and taking the appropriate vitamin supplements a heart friendly diet can go a long way to reversing plaque build-up. The easy part is that it's the same diet that I've mentioned throughout this book. Consuming lots of green vegetables, fruits that have a low glycaemic index such as apples, pears, pawpaw, cherries and all the berry fruits, eating less bread, breakfast cereal, rice, potato and pasta, substituting the smaller fish and white meat for red meat, cooking with small amounts of extra-virgin olive oil, consuming tempeh if you're a vegetarian and having regular snacks of seeds and nuts especially almonds and cashews is the ideal way to terminate any recalcitrant plaque that is lingering in your blood vessels. If you add a regular exercise regime, which includes maintaining a sweat for a least 40-50minutes five times a week and this would mean either jogging, riding a pushbike or walking briskly, then your plaque will simply have nowhere to hide.

ANTIOXIDANTS, HERBAL MEDICINES AND ASSORTED NUTRIENTS

Flavonoids are a group of compounds with antioxidant properties that are found in large quantities in apples, onions, broccoli, cocoa products, red grapes and tea. Although I'm not a great endorser of chocolate and alcohol consumption the good news for those who enjoy this pastime is that dark chocolate and not more than 1-2 glasses of red wine daily have a wide range of anti-inflammatory, antioxidant and potentially blood pressure lowering benefits. My preference is to suggest you take 5mg of the concentrated form of red grape extract or resveratrol daily. Tea lovers are also winners as five cups per day of black tea over a three-week period has been shown to reduce total cholesterol by 6.5%, LDL (by) 11.1%, apolipoprotein B (by) 5% and lipoprotein (a) (by) 16.4%.

SOY

For the knockers of soy 50grams per day of soy protein has been shown to reduce total cholesterol and LDL. Soy can also reduce homocysteine and prevent LDL from becoming oxidised.

POLICOSANOL

Policosanol is a substance derived from sugar cane extract. Clinical trials conducted over 24 weeks have demonstrated that 20mg per day and 40mg per day lowered LDL by 27.4% and 28.1% and total cholesterol by 15.6% and 17.3% respectively. Interestingly in the 20mg group HDL went up by 17.6% whereas the 40mg group experienced less of a benefit with their HDL only improving by 17%. (31) Policosanol also has the ability to inhibit the oxidation of LDL and to protect the endothelium. In one study this substance was shown to lead to regression of plaque accumulation in a small group of subjects. (32)

OMEGA-3 FATTY ACIDS

Omega-3 fatty acids found predominantly in fatty fish including salmon, tuna, mackerel, sardines and herring and here the latter three smaller fish would be your best bet, as the mercury content of these is likely to be minimal, protect your endothelium, make your heart beat regularly if you are suffering from an irregular heart rhythm, decrease triglycerides, another dangerous fat that you want to restrict, and even prevent vulnerable plaque from rupturing making this a highly valuable nutrient for the health of your heart.

So that vegetarians don't feel hard done by, flaxseed is also a useful source of omega-3 fatty acids although it has to be said that this vegetable source of omega-3 fatty acids is not as potent as that which is derived from fish.   1-2 dessertspoons of ground flaxseeds taken daily would be a better option than flaxseed oil and 1-2 grams of fish oil would provide a therapeutic dose of omega-3 fatty acids.

COENZYME Q10

I'm a great fan of coenzyme Q10 as it has encouraging antioxidant and energy boosting potential and works in unison with vitamins C and E as well as alpha-lipoic acid to enhance the potency of these nutrients.   Coenzyme Q10 has been shown to improve heart muscle function, lower blood pressure, reduce free radical stress and increase HDL levels, which is a nice little quartet of benefits.   The statin medications used to lower cholesterol reduce the liver's production of coenzyme Q10 which might be one of the reasons for the side-effects of these medications including muscle pain, impairment of heart muscle function, memory loss and elevation of liver enzymes. With American authorities indicating that we should be aiming for even lower

LDL levels to prevent heart disease or to protect those who have already had a heart attack and with the emergence of more powerful statin drugs to achieve these ends the potential to diminish the protective advantage of coenzymeQ10 is increasing. There is no doubt that statins can substantially reduce inflammation and LDL, improve the prognosis of those who suffer from heart disease, stabilise and even gobble up plaque. If you are taking one of the statin medications then including coenzymeQ10 might help to limit the side-effects of these drugs.

There are a vast array of other natural substances which have cholesterol and LDL lowering effects including ground flaxseed, psyllium seeds, oats, avocado, barley, walnuts, magnesium, olive oil and phytosterols incorporated in margarines. These might not be as effective as statins but together with all the other remedies I've mentioned might form just as formidable an army against heart disease without any adverse consequences.

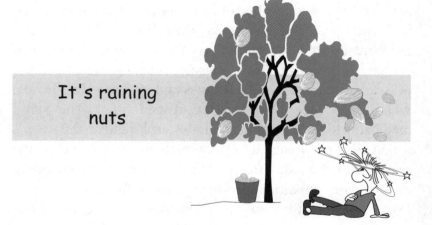

It's raining nuts

This is how you can go about preventing heart disease.

- Limit your consumption of red meat, dairy products, eggs and refined carbohydrates
- Eat healthy amounts of green vegetables, nuts, flaxseeds, apples, onions, garlic and berry fruits
- Drink black and green tea
- Consume ginger and turmeric
- Deal appropriately with emotional stress
- Exercise regularly
- Maintain optimal weight
- See that your blood pressure stays around 115/75
- Boost your liver function with herbs such as globe artichoke, dandelion and st mary's thistle
- Limit homocysteine, lipoprotein (a) and inflammation
- Maintain optimal levels of HDL
- Reduce LDL especially small, dense LDL and oxidised LDL
- Limit cholesterol and triglycerides
- Maintain optimal levels of oestrogen and progesterone for women
- Preserve optimal levels of thyroid hormone for both sexes
- Take inositol hexanicotinate and/or policosanol to increase HDL and lower cholesterol if necessary
- Take vitamin E in the form of mixed tocopherols and tocotrienols
- Take vitamin C, coenzyme Q10 and omega-3 fatty acids either in the form of fish oil or ground flaxseeds

LOOKING AFTER YOUR BRAIN

It's so easy to look after your brain if you're taking all the steps that we've already gone through to prevent heart disease. The very same processes that lead to heart disease also compromise your brain function. Free radical excess, the accumulation of plaque, inflammation, ongoing emotional and work stress, elevated homocysteine and lipoprotein (a), raised blood pressure, exposure to cigarette smoke and uncontrolled blood sugar, all factors with which you are highly familiar by now will lead to the progressive erosion of your higher powers and even possibly Alzheimer's and Parkinson's disease. Stroke is almost certainly caused by these events. Once you're neutralising these destructive forces you're going a long way to preserving your mental function.

Your brain is a highly active organ. It uses 20% of the total energy expended by your body to carry out its daily function. This is also the problem. The more energy that your cells use the greater the generation of free radicals, which makes your brain highly vulnerable. The cells of your brain are encased in a layer of fat like an insulation process, which protects them. But fat can go rancid. This means that your brain cells are faced with a double whammy. Ever increasing free radicals that are poised to wreak destructive havoc and oodles of fat that can easily become rotten and decayed. This is why it is so important to be extremely solicitous with regard to the health of your brain.

What most of us are concerned about when we realise that our mental functions are going into decline is our memories. It's normal for your memory to become less sharp as you get older. However if you're regularly struggling to remember where you put things, you're constantly having difficulty recalling people's names after you've been introduced and you just can't seem to remember the name of that famous actress then this is cause for some concern. The loss of short-term memory is one of the first signs of Alzheimer's disease. There's no doubt that we have to put more effort into remembering, as we get older. However, if you can recollect the events that took place thirty years ago with crystal clarity and what happened yesterday is a murky haze then you might have to pay extra special attention to the segment on Alzheimer's disease coming up shortly. What is for certain is that we could all do with enhanced powers of remembering. If you want to boost your memory here's how you can go about doing this.

THE HORMONES

OESTROGEN

In theory oestrogen is highly beneficial for women. Oestrogen is a powerful antioxidant with the ability to stimulate memory function, promote the growth of new nerves and protect the brain. There is even evidence that oestrogen causes the breakdown of the harmful protein that leads to Alzheimer's disease. (33) Oestrogen equips female rats with better memories and makes them more adaptable when exposed to ongoing stress whereas male animals fall apart in similar conditions. (34) This makes it easier to appreciate why females find it so easy to do so many things at once while us mere mortals struggle to watch television and drink beer at the same time. If you're feeling depressed, mentally foggy and increasingly forgetful, especially if you're going through the menopausal transition, these symptoms could be due to low oestrogen levels. Correct this imbalance and your old bright and sunny disposition might resurface.

Unfortunately, when it comes to examining the scientific evidence there are studies which show that oestrogen improves memory and mental function while there are others that don't report these benefits. (35) (36) (37) The Women's Health Initiative trial which examined whether oestrogen could improve memory and prevent dementia in a large group of 65-79 year-old women found exactly the opposite, that taking oestrogen actually diminished cognitive function. (38) How do you make sense out of all this and should you consider boosting your oestrogen levels or avoiding this hormone?

As I've already indicated all the negative findings emanating from the Women's Health Initiative trial probably resulted from the administration of the wrong type of hormones at an inopportune time in these women's lives. Canadian expert Dr Barbara Sherwin, who has written an extensive review on this subject, suggests that the critical period for commencing oestrogen treatment is in the immediate postmenopausal period. She indicates that you might have the greatest chance for preventing cognitive decline and Alzheimer's disease by starting oestrogen during this time. (39)

Although the jury is still out on this issue I'm going to go with Dr Sherwin's findings and propose that if your oestrogen levels are low utilizing triest, the combination of the three oestrogens, or oestradiol on its own might give you the mental edge that you need as well as affording you some protection against the development of Alzheimer's disease. It also might be helpful to observe that 5-day hormone-free period each month. If you constantly bombard your oestrogen receptors with stimulation they can become unresponsive and you will lose the benefits of oestrogen.

PROGESTERONE

Progesterone has traditionally been thought of as a hormone which stills the mind and dulls the memory. However, collaborative research between Argentinean and French scientists intimates that this hormone has regenerative capabilities and might be useful for preserving cognitive function during ageing. Indeed, animal studies demonstrate that progesterone can promote the regrowth of myelin, the protective coating which is vital for the function of nerve fibres. (40) Depending on your levels anywhere from 20-40mg of progesterone cream applied at night or 200-400mg of the troche would be appropriate.

TESTOSTERONE

Testosterone levels can go into decline with ageing, which might be responsible for memory loss and the deterioration of all the other mental functions over time. Like oestrogen for women testosterone offers the promise of a whole range of cognitive advantages for men. Testosterone enhances blood flow to those areas of the brain responsible for reasoning and memory and stimulates the growth of nerve cells. (41) (42) Intriguingly, many of the benefits of testosterone might have a lot to do with its conversion to oestrogen. The incidence of Alzheimer's disease is far lower in men and this might be due to the presence of a larger reservoir of testosterone that can be used to manufacture protective oestrogen. Testosterone appears to enhance the visual side of memory while oestrogen makes it easier for men to put things into words. (43)

One study found that men with prostate cancer who received treatment to suppress testosterone found it that much harder to remember compared with those men who had healthy levels of this hormone. Another indicates that higher levels of testosterone lead to better memories. (44)

If your testosterone levels are low and your mental powers are diminishing then augmenting your supplies of this hormone might be worthwhile and might provide you with some protection against developing Alzheimer's disease and the other dementias that occur with ageing. 25-50mg of testosterone cream applied daily or a similar dose in troche form would be therapeutic.

GROWTH HORMONE

The production of growth hormone and its partner IGF-1 also subside with ageing. As is the case with oestrogen and testosterone, IGF-1 has numerous positive effects on brain function by promoting nerve growth factors, preserving the integrity of the hippocampus, that part of the brain responsible for memory function, encouraging the growth of new blood vessels which feed ailing brain cells and helping to clear beta-amyloid, the toxic protein associated with Alzheimer's disease. (45) It's also interesting to remember that both oestrogen and testosterone used topically can increase IGF-1 levels. Higher IGF-1 levels have been associated with improved performance on tests of cognition in older men while lower levels predicted cognitive decline. (46)

If blood tests do show that you are lacking in IGF-1 and your mental functions are diminishing then you have a number of options. Boosting oestrogen or testosterone if these are low might be useful. Taking secretagogues, which increase growth hormone such as the combination of glycine, glutamine and niacin detailed in chapter two or trans-D tropin is another possibility. (47) Failing these, growth hormone injections would be another alternative.

DEHYDROEPIANDROSTERONE (DHEA)

DHEA has a wide range of neuroprotective and neurotrophic effects. It has the ability to salvage those parts of the brain responsible for memory, stimulate nerve growth and shelter brain cells from the destructive effects of the stress hormone cortisol. Remember that DHEA is also the hormone that is the principal source for making oestrogen and testosterone. There are a number of animal studies which testify to the benefits of DHEA on memory and cognitive ability in ageing animals. Although human trials have been less consistent in demonstrating any positive effects of DHEA on memory there is a study which shows that this hormone has antidepressant and memory boosting potential. (48)

The same strategy that applies to the hormones mentioned above would equally apply to DHEA. If your levels are low, especially if your cortisol levels are elevated, then taking 10-25mg of DHEA cream daily might provide you with additional cognitive support.

PREGNENOLONE

Pregnenolone is another hormone that has been shown to offset age-related memory deficits in animals. This hormone is also thought to protect the nerve cells of the brain. Human trials have yet to confirm these findings. Although this is somewhat conjectural 100mg of pregnenolone taken orally might provide you with some memory benefits.

THYROID HORMONES

Thyroid hormones are vitally important for the function of your brain. If your thyroid hormones are not serving you adequately you will become sluggish and slow and your memory and cognitive ability will be significantly impaired. Thyroid treatment in those who do not produce sufficient amounts of thyroid hormone has been shown to improve memory. This would be a good time to review thyroid hormone management described in chapter two.

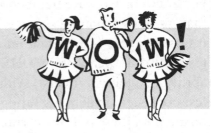

Go Hormones

All your hormones work in tandem to preserve your cognitive powers and to protect you from the ravages of neurodegenerative diseases such as Alzheimer's and Parkinson's disease. If your hormone levels are low then taking all the appropriate measures to optimise these might provide you with the mental sustenance you need to improve dwindling memory resources.

THE VITAMINS

If hormones give memory processes a boost then vitamins are the fuel which maintains the brain's vital powers. Acetylcholine, the neurotransmitter which is responsible for the activation and consolidation of memory, depends upon B vitamins for its synthesis. Learning difficulties, fatigue, depression, memory problems and even dementia are all tied in with B vitamin deficiencies. Homocysteine (the toxic protein that leads to heart disease) has also been associated with the development of Alzheimer's disease and the onset of strokes. Having adequate supplies of vitamins B6, B12 and folic acid is one way to render homocysteine relatively harmless. It is not difficult to slip into B vitamin deficit. Stress is probably the largest B vitamin drain. Then there's alcohol, caffeine, hormone treatments containing oestrogen, antacid medications, vegetarian diets and the heating of foods. As you get older your body's ability to absorb vitamin B12 becomes increasingly compromised. Taking medications that suppress your body's production of acid by the stomach, which is sadly what older folk are often given when they complain of digestive upsets, will make it even harder to get the vitamin B12 you need. Many of the patients I see, especially those with fatigue, moodiness and loss of memory, are simply lacking in vitamin B12. Meat, fish, eggs, green vegetables, brown rice, tofu, nuts and sunflower seeds are good sources of B vitamins.

Along with the B vitamins, vitamins C, D, E and beta-carotene have all been linked with enhanced cognitive ability and the prevention of dementia.

I was especially heartened by a study conducted by a group of Canadian research scientists at McMaster University in Hamilton, Ontario in which they showed that a dietary supplement containing hormones, vitamins and antioxidants, the principal ingredients being the B group vitamins, beta-carotene, vitamins C, D and E, coenzyme Q10, DHEA, melatonin and gingko biloba was able to abolish age-related cognitive decline and rejuvenate learning and memory in a group of ageing mice. The authors of this research claimed that the formulation was able to achieve these outcomes by increasing insulin sensitivity and glucose utilisation, reducing inflammation, limiting free radical stress and improving the function of the mitochondria, the batteries driving cellular energy. (49) This is the very point I'm at pains to emphasize. It is the combination of the right nutrients that operate as a team rather than individual supplements used in isolation that appears to have the strongest ability to curb the processes that lead to brain ageing.

To get the maximum benefits from all the vitamins mentioned above you need the following taken daily:

- Vitamins B1, B2 and B3 100mg of each
- Vitamin B12 500mcg
- Folic acid 400mcg
- Beta-carotene 10mg
- Vitamin C 1gram
- Vitamin E 400mg of mixed tocopherols together with 50mg of mixed tocotrienols
- Vitamin D 1000i.u.

THE DIET

The brain thrives on the same diet that is good for the heart. Green vegetables such as broccoli, spinach, Brussels sprouts, cabbage and cauliflower, low glycaemic index fruits including apples, pears, pawpaw, cherries and all the berry fruits, organically grown if possible, the good fats found in extra-virgin olive oil, avocado, nuts and seeds and protein in chicken, turkey, lean red meat (all preferably free-range and organically fed) together with tempeh, beans, chickpeas and lentils would provide your brain with all the essential elements of a healthy diet. The omega-3 fatty acids located in small fish such as sardines, orange roughie, haddock and perch (which are likely to have minimal mercury content) as well as flaxseed, contain the vital nutrient docosahexaenoic acid (DHA) which has been shown to improve cognitive function and protect the hippocampus, the memory centre of the brain. By reducing inflammation, making blood flow more easily and preventing harmful fats from accumulating DHA is thought to have a major role in limiting those events that contribute to cognitive decline with ageing. If your preference is to incorporate flaxseeds rather than fish because you are a vegetarian or for any other reason, then you need to ensure that you have adequate supplies of zinc and magnesium as you need these nutrients to convert omega-3 fatty acids to DHA. This process is slightly less efficient in generating DHA than the fish option. Zinc containing foods are sunflower and pumpkin seeds, ginger, beans and peas while green vegetables and nuts are rich sources of magnesium.

While you are loading up on the beneficial fats it is just as worthwhile limiting the fats that are less nourishing of your brain cells and these would include red meat, whole-fat dairy products and the trans fatty acids found in fried foods and margarines which make your cell membranes less flexible and receptive.

Then you have to ensure that you don't have any food intolerances. I have found that gluten found in wheat, rye, oats and barley as well as yeast-rich foods such as vegemite, bread and mushrooms are common offenders. As well as being associated with digestive complaints like burping, bloating and gas these can also gum up your mental processes leading to a lack of mental clarity and memory impairment. Simple blood tests, which measure gliadin and candida antibodies, can identify gluten and yeast intolerance respectively. Then it's simply a matter of avoiding gluten if you turn up a positive blood test and/or treating yeast or candida overgrowth according to the principles laid out in chapter two if this is your problem.

Finally there are the memory boosters like blueberries and spinach, which make rats much sharper and might just do the same for us humans. Blueberries even have the ability to increase the production of new nerve cells in the hippocampus where memories are consolidated and what's more these little wonders of nature can facilitate the formation of those nerve pathways that allow for the transfer of memory traces from short to long-term memory.

THE SPECIAL NUTRIENTS

ACETYL-L-CARNITINE AND ALPHA-LIPOIC ACID

Once you are on the above diet and taking the vitamins which can help to energise your mental functions you can also invest in a number of potentially cognitive enhancing nutrients. A nice little animal study on ageing rats has shown that the combination of acetyl-L-carnitine, which helps to shuttle fats into the mitochondria where they are used for energy, and alpha-lipoic acid (the multitasking antioxidant) improved memory, revitalised energy, reduced free radical damage to the hippocampus, the memory centre of the brain and generally rejuvenated the mental capacity of these elder statesmen.

Although we don't yet have human trials which substantiate these benefits, if these nutrients can help ageing rats they might well be able save us. Like many other experts who embrace the promise of these studies I'm going to suggest that it might be advantageous to include acetyl-L-carnitine and alpha-lipoic acid in your medicine chest.

GINGKO BILOBA

Gingko biloba is the oldest surviving deciduous tree on earth and therefore it is not surprising that this herb has a multitude of healthful qualities including antioxidant and anti-inflammatory capabilities. Aside from enriching mental function gingko also plays a part in relieving anxiety and stress, managing tinnitus, improving circulation and even treating erectile dysfunction. Gingko is especially useful for treating those already suffering from diminished cognitive capacity. Dementia and Alzheimer's sufferers and those afflicted with a syndrome known as cerebral insufficiency which results in difficulties with concentration and memory as well as absent-mindedness and ongoing mental confusion have been shown to have clearly discernable mental improvements when taking gingko.

The question is, can gingko make it easier for those of us who do not experience severe cognitive impairments to engage our memories? This is where the results are conflicting. One study recorded in the Journal of the American Medical Association (50) revealed that over a six-week period healthy adults experienced no benefits with regard to memory when taking gingko biloba compared with a placebo group. Other studies on both elderly and young adults have demonstrated just the opposite, that gingko does boost memory. It is possible to argue that six weeks is not long enough to derive any gains from gingko or you could invoke the notion that gingko only makes an impression once you are demonstrably mentally compromised. My suggestion is not to wait until your mental faculties are deserting you before investing in gingko.

BACOPA MONNIERA (BRAHMI)

Bacopa monniera also known as brahmi has been an important part of the Ayurvedic tradition since the sixth century A.D. It has been used to improve memory and concentration and to facilitate learning. Current scientific evidence does support this with a clinical trial proving that brahmi 300mg enhanced cognitive performance and boosted memory in a group of healthy adults over a 12 week period. (51) Brahmi is another herb that you can consider adding to your brain boosting strategy.

PHOSPHATIDYLSERINE

If stress is your nemesis then phosphatidylserine could be your saviour. This nutrient, which is derived from soy, has the ability to suppress the release of the stress hormone cortisol and this has the effect of limiting the damaging effects of this hormone on the hippocampus. Phosphatidylserine also protects cell membranes, which allows brain cells to communicate with each other and relay information more efficiently. One trial conducted in the USA has demonstrated that phosphatidylserine was able to rejuvenate memory by a whopping 14 years in a group of 50-70 year old men and women suffering from memory loss. (52) Significant improvements were noted with remembering names after introduction, which is an advantage we all could use, as well as the capacity to dial a 10-digit telephone number from memory, another significant benefit. Phosphatidylserine also has antioxidant properties, which is an added bonus as the effects of free radical overload can escalate with ageing.

VINCA MINOR AND VINPOCETINE

Vinca minor is a herb which improves cerebral blood flow, increases the rate at which the brain produces energy and speeds up the use of glucose and oxygen in the brain. All these benefits have been harnessed to help manage a range of conditions including stroke, vertigo, tinnitus, Meniere's disease, epilepsy and cerebral insufficiency or poor circulation to the brain. Vinpocetine is the synthetic derivative of vinca minor, which has been shown to benefit short-term memory but has really come into its own when used to treat dementia sufferers. Clinical trials have confirmed that this nutrient has been particularly effective for improving memory and attention span in this group of patients.

CARNOSINE

Another nutrient, which has been touted as the next best thing with regard to limiting the ageing process is carnosine. One of the factors that contributes to ageing is the accumulation of sugars in the bloodstream which coat cellular protein leading to the formation of what is aptly termed AGEs or advanced glycosylation end products. This would be similar to the accumulation of rust that progressively corrodes the metal pipes of your house. The shortening of telomeres, which exist at the end of chromosomes, is another primary event that limits the capacity of cells to replicate thereby promoting ageing. Carnosine's prospects lie in its ability to interrupt both of these ageing processes. Carnosine has antioxidant, membrane stabilising and chelating properties, which allows this nutrient to remove heavy metal poisons such as lead, aluminium and mercury from the body. These qualities suggest that carnosine is ideally suited to protect ageing brains and to support this notion there are animal studies intimating that this nutrient could be useful to prevent and treat stroke. Although carnosine has helped to improve the behaviour and communication skills of autistic children there aren't any studies yet proving that our memories or mental powers will be enhanced by this nutrient.

Like the other nutrients mentioned above the ability that carnosine might have to put the shackles on the forces that erode our mental powers is what makes carnosine appealing. You can get your carnosine from red meat or you can opt to take supplements if you want to obtain what appears to be a healthy protective advantage from this substance.

ALPHA-GLYCERYLPHOSPHORYLCHOLINE

Alpha-glycerylphosphorylcholine is a substance derived from soy that your brain can utilise to make more acetylcholine, the brain chemical that facilitates memory. A commonly held belief amongst scientists is that nerve cells are deprived of this essential chemical with ageing which in turn leads to memory loss and the other typical features of cognitive decline. Provide a ready source of acetylcholine and cognitive ageing can be reversed. This might be a tad simplistic but once again there are those trusty animal studies showing that alpha-glycerylphosphorylcholine is able to increase acetylcholine levels and boost the learning and memory capacity of ageing rats.

Then there are the trials, which investigated the effects of alpha-glycerylphosphorylcholine on those patients with dementia, Alzheimer's disease and stroke, consistently demonstrating clinical improvements in memory and cognitive performance. Alpha-glycerylphosphorylcholine even has the ability to increase growth hormone levels. If animals and dementia sufferers can benefit should we all be supplementing with this nutrient to combat memory loss and brain ageing? The optimists would answer in the affirmative while the sceptics would require more evidence. I believe that our brains need every bit of help they can get and therefore my inclination is to endorse alpha-glycerylphosphorylcholine and to encourage you to supplement with this nutrient.

SOY

There's no doubt about it. Controversy follows soy like honey captivates the bee. If you're a soy consumer you'll embrace all the studies showing that this substance boosts memory and is beneficial for your brain. Unfortunately there is also evidence that tofu which is made from soy is associated with dementia. This was a study performed on Hawaiian males which revealed that the more tofu the males consumed the greater the incidence of dementia. (53) To add further support to the possible harm that soy might be inflicting an experiment which involved adding soy to a tissue culture of brain cells demonstrated that this nutrient blocked the formation of new brain cells and exposed those present to increasing levels of toxicity. The brains of male rats have also been found to shrivel up when exposed to soy. Fascinatingly the opposite seems to happen to female rats suggesting that soy might be protective to female brains.

When it comes to human studies some show that soy is the tonic that female brains thrive on while others reveal that soy doesn't improve cognitive function in women. (54) (55) If you want to add further confusion to the mix, a detailed review of all soy's benefits points out that this nutrient does have antioxidant and anti-inflammatory effects, which is something our ageing brains could really use. (56) Before the fellow vegetarians and soy consumers decide to abandon this substance which might make finding an alternative source of protein rather difficult my suggestion is to consume mostly fermented soy in the form of tempeh and to limit your intake to 3-4 times weekly.

Here then is a list of all the nutrients that might enhance your memory and protect your brain together with their daily doses:

- Alpha-lipoic acid 200mg
- Acetyl-L-carnitine 500mg
- Gingko biloba 120mg of the standard extract
- Bacopa monniera (Brahmi) 100mg of the standard extract
- Phosphatidylserine 100mg
- Vinca minor 80mg of the standard extract
- Carnosine 1000mg
- Alpha-glycerylphosphorylcholine 1200mg

Aside from putting all the right nutrients in your mouth there are a host of other strategies you can adopt to ensure that your brain gets all the help it needs. There is a chapter called 'Boosting Brain Power' in my first book 'Eternal health' which details these and there is also a very useful section in Dr Perlmutter's 'Better Brain Book' listing all the exercises you can adopt to maintain good mental function. Essentially you need to constantly challenge your brain and remain mentally active. You need to practice remembering. If you're a visual person using unusual images will help you to recall the names of people you've just met. Auditory learners can utilise repetitive sounds to help form permanent mental imprints.

Finally a few words about the long-term use of mobile phones. I'm probably the only person who doesn't have one. Everybody is using them and sometimes the conversations can be somewhat protracted. This is disturbing as there is evidence, which associates this practice with the development of brain cancer. Reassuringly there is also a Danish study, which failed to establish any connection between the use of cellular telephones and the risk of developing acoustic neuroma, a form of brain cancer.

If you do need your mobile phone my advice is to restrict your conversation time to the bare minimum and for those who desire added protection, which would be a wise investment based on current practices, taking gingko biloba might be the way to go. A study on a group of animals who were exposed to electro magnetic irradiation similar to that which is emitted by mobile phones found that this herb preserved those antioxidants responsible for nullifying any adverse free radical damage that mobile phones might generate.

PREVENTING AND TREATING ALZHEIMER'S DISEASE

Alzheimer's is a harrowing disease. I had a patient once, a highly gifted pianist, and her husband who had to witness the relentless ebbing of her mental faculties used to remind me regularly about the bright and highly intelligent woman she used to be. If it's any consolation sufferers of this disease appear to be unaware of the progressive erosion of their cognitive powers. It's their carers who have to cope with the ordeal of watching their loved ones slowly disappear in front of their eyes. There is no cure for Alzheimer's disease but new treatments are emerging that can ameliorate symptoms and slow the evolution of this disease. There is also no definitive diagnostic test available yet which unequivocally establishes the presence of Alzheimer's disease.   It's really the typical symptoms that suggest this terrible form of dementia is setting in.

The earliest discernible symptom is short-term memory loss, which becomes increasingly pervasive so that it becomes more difficult to remember what happened the day before or that the relatives actually did visit last week   Interestingly loss of the sense of smell predates this symptom by at least two years. Once memory loss is established Alzheimer's sufferers start to find it difficult to perform routine tasks like switching on the washing machine or turning off the stove.   Self-expression becomes limited and mood changes such as irritability, depression and irrationality become a regular feature.   This then leads to confusion, disorientation and wandering at all hours of the night.   Inevitably there is an inexorable regression to a state of infantile dependency.

By the time you reach 65 you will have a 10% chance of developing Alzheimer's and this escalates dramatically with ageing so that celebrating your 85th birthday also carries with it a 50% possibility of succumbing to this affliction. Now this might not be an especially comforting notion but the good news is that there is a lot you can do to protect yourself against the development of this condition. Although we don't yet have the final handle on all those factors that result in the development of Alzheimer's we do have a fair idea of the precipitating events that trigger this disease. It all revolves around the excessive accumulation of a substance called amyloid beta protein in the brain. We all have this protein but those who develop Alzheimer's disease appear to accumulate a whole lot more of amyloid beta protein. Free radical excess and inflammation, two familiar foes, are the driving forces that boost amyloid beta protein build-up. If you then add to the mix a diet rich in saturated fats found in red meat and dairy products, trans fats in margarines and fried foods, elevated homocysteine and cholesterol levels, the presence of aluminium, iron, copper and zinc, repeated head injuries, the deposition of sugar coated proteins called AGEs and a gene called ApoE4 that increases your risk then you have all the major players involved in the ongoing promotion of amyloid beta protein and the increasing destruction of your brain cells.

What's reassuring about all this is that for the most part all these precipitating events can be measured with the appropriate tests and even prevented. Free radical excess can be evaluated by means of the biological terrain assessment test, which I'll describe in the final chapter or by utilising the organix urine profile including the quantification of a substance known as 8-hydroxy-2'-deoxyguanosine that measures oxidative or free radical damage to DNA. Inflammation is simply calculated by doing a blood test, which examines your HS-CRP levels. A blood test can also measure your cholesterol and homocysteine levels while glucose or sugar metabolism can be assessed by way of doing fasting blood glucose and insulin assay and repeating these at the hourly and 2 hourly mark. Elevated glucose levels will indicate that your metabolism of this substance is inefficient which means you will have extra amounts of glucose travelling around your bloodstream that can then attach to protein molecules to form the damaging compound AGEs. The presence of iron, copper, aluminium and zinc can be appraised by doing a hair mineral analysis which involves cutting some hair from the back of your head close to the roots and sending this to a laboratory in the USA for testing.

Once you have all this information you can then take the necessary steps to deal with any abnormalities that show up on your tests. Whilst doing this is not an absolute guarantee that you won't get Alzheimer's disease at least you'll be going some of the way to minimising those harmful processes that contribute to the advancement of this awful condition. Here's how you can employ hormones, vitamins, diet and special nutrients to protect yourself.

THE HORMONES
OESTROGEN

On paper oestrogen has all the smarts to prevent Alzheimer's disease. Oestradiol, which is the strongest oestrogen, prevents the accumulation of beta-amyloid, the protein associated with Alzheimer's. Starting oestradiol replacement soon after menopause when levels of this hormone start to wain appears to be the ideal way to benefit from the protective effects of oestradiol with regard to preventing Alzheimer's disease, which is why the Women's Health Initiative Memory study failed to demonstrate that hormone replacement was of any use. In my previous comments on this study, which showed that commencing hormone replacement more that 10 years after menopause does not improve memory and in fact leads to higher rates of dementia, I've indicated that this approach simply constitutes the application of the wrong type of hormone treatment when it is already too late. If you allow yourself to become oestrogen deficient after menopause by waiting for 10 years before you start taking hormones then you might not be able to take advantage of the many protective benefits of oestradiol.

PROGESTERONE

Progesterone potentiates the neuroprotective effects of oestrogen whereas medroxyprogesterone acetate which is the progestogen found in Provera does exactly the opposite. Combining progesterone with oestrogen might be the ideal way to protect female brains.

TESTOSTERONE

One reason for the decrease in the incidence of Alzheimer's disease in the male sex is thought to be related to our ability to use testosterone to make oestrogen. Having more testosterone enables us to manufacture protective oestrogen, which the female sex would not be able to do as they get older due to extremely limited testosterone resources. Testosterone in its own right can reduce beta amyloid and protect the male brain independently of its conversion to oestrogen. It's not surprising then that low testosterone levels are associated with Alzheimer's disease. What is extremely encouraging is a study which shows that men with higher free testosterone levels appear to have a reduced risk of developing Alzheimer's disease. (57) The authors of this research are of the opinion that maintaining testosterone in the upper part of the normal range may be the fortification that men need against Alzheimer's disease. Although there aren't studies yet which show that taking testosterone prevents Alzheimer's it would appear to make some sense to consider augmenting your supplies of this hormone if your levels are low.

DHEA

In a German study low DHEA has been associated with the development of Alzheimer's disease. (58) The same principles that apply to the other hormones can be invoked here. If your levels of DHEA are low taking extra DHEA might just help to prevent Alzheimer's disease.

MELATONIN

If free radical stress promotes Alzheimer's disease then melatonin, which is the hormone with wide-ranging antioxidant properties, might be one of your body's major weapons against the advancement of this disease. Checking your levels via salivary hormone assays and supplementing if these are low might provide you with another string in your bow to ward of this neurodegenerative condition.

THE VITAMINS

Vitamins C and E are the major contenders here. An American study has indicated that taking vitamin E 400i.u together with vitamin C 500mg was able to reduce the incidence of Alzheimer's disease by a whopping 78%. (59) Taking extra Niacin or vitamin B3 might also be a wise investment as evidenced by an American report indicating that those individuals who consumed foods rich in this nutrient had a lesser chance of developing Alzheimer's. I still believe that it would be worthwhile protecting yourself with a combination of nutrients rather than relying on individual vitamins to provide you with the fortification you need.

THE DIET

Omega-3 fatty acids found in fish, flaxseed and nuts as well as blueberries and apples are the magical substances that have been shown to reduce the risk of Alzheimer's disease. Following a group of participants for over four years research scientists discovered that the crucial nutrient preventing the development of Alzheimer's disease was omega-3 fatty acids. (60) Although the evidence for the protective effects of blueberries was generated by animal studies the potential of blueberries to safeguard our brains cannot be disputed. Apples, which are a major source of quercetin, another antioxidant which can protect our brains from the damaging effects of free radicals, might also provide a possible buffer against Alzheimer's disease.   If you then add to these nutrients the healthy diet described in detail on page 274 you will be taking significant steps to minimise your risk of developing Alzheimer's disease.

THE SPECIAL NUTRIENTS

Alpha-lipoic acid, coenzyme Q10 and carnosine are all lining up to intercept those factors that induce Alzheimer's disease. The combined abilities of these nutrients to recycle other antioxidants, neutralise free radicals and inhibit the aggregation of Beta-amyloid is impressive. The anti-inflammatory herb curcumin, which can also bind heavy metals, together with gotu kola which has been shown to reduce free radical stress, can be utilised with the many talents of ginkgo biloba to arrest the development of Alzheimer's disease.

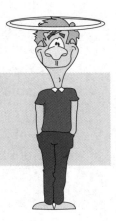

I'm a Special Nutrient

While the evidence is preliminary, here are the hormones and nutrients that taken together daily might prevent Alzheimer's disease. Oestradiol, testosterone, DHEA and melatonin should only be incorporated once you've had your levels measured and they are low.

- Oestradiol cream or troches ½-1mg or Triest cream or troches 1-2mg for women
- Testosterone cream or troches 25-50mg for men
- DHEA cream 15mg for women
- DHEA cream 25mg for men
- Melatonin 1-3mg orally at night
- Vitamin C 500mg
- Vitamin E 400 i.u comprising mixed tocopherols and 50mg of the mixed tocotrienols.
- Niacin 500mg
- Omega-3 fatty acids 1 gram
- Alpha-lipoic acid 200mg
- Coenzyme Q10 200mg
- Carnosine 500mg
- Curcumin 200mg
- Ginkgo biloba 120mg
- Gotu kola 100mg

TREATING ALZHEIMER'S DISEASE

Right now our capacity to treat Alzheimer's disease is limited. However, of all the medications used to manage this disorder, the drug memantine, which limits free radical production, has the most potential to make inroads on the progression of this disease. Then there are the hormonal interventions along with nutritional supplements and herbal medicines that have been shown to ameliorate the symptoms of Alzheimer's sufferers.

THE HORMONES
OESTROGEN

The studies using horse oestrogen failed to show that this hormone had any influence on the mental or behavioural function of Alzheimer's sufferers. On the positive side, when oestrogen was administered in the form of a low dose oestradiol cream clear improvements in memory were demonstrated. The oestrogen treatment also made it easier for this group of women to look after themselves and decreased their level of disorientation. (61) (62)

TESTOSTERONE

Despite the evidence that testosterone boosts memory and cognitive ability, especially for those men who are low in this hormone, there haven't been many studies exploring the benefits of testosterone on Alzheimer's disease. One small study on a group of males who had reduced levels of testosterone indicated that treatment with this hormone did improve mental function while the placebo group who did not receive any testosterone deteriorated gradually. (63)

MELATONIN

Alzheimer's leads to disruptions of the sleep-wake cycle so that sufferers of this disease become agitated towards sundown and tend to get up and wander at all hours of the night. Melatonin can restore normal circadian rhythms, which makes it easier to establish regular and more restful sleep patterns. Melatonin is also a very effective antioxidant, which might help to combat the free radical processes that drive Alzheimer's disease.

THE SPECIAL NUTRIENTS

Both ginkgo biloba and vitamin E in high doses have been shown to improve memory and cognitive performance as well as slow the progression of Alzheimer's disease. Nicotinamide adenine dinucleotide (NADH), a substance which plays a vital role in the energy production of the cell, also helps to enhance mental function in patients with Alzheimer's disease. In one study a group of patients who took 10mg of NADH orally for six months had a superior performance on a number of tests, which evaluated verbal performance and abstract thinking compared with another group who received a placebo.

Acetyl-L-carnitine is another substance, which reduces cognitive impairment when it is used in the early stages of Alzheimer's disease. Acetyl-L-carnitine has the ability to enhance the efficacy of conventional medications used to manage Alzheimer's disease so that with the addition of this substance significant improvements have been noted in cognitive functioning and behaviour.

Huperzia serrata also known as huperzine, a herb that has been used in Traditional Chinese Medicine because of its circulation boosting and anti-inflammatory properties, has been shown to increase acetylcholine (the brain chemical which enhances memory) and to protect brain cells from the toxic effects of beta-amyloid. In one trial huperzine substantially improved memory and behaviour in Alzheimer's patients. (64)

The herb lemon balm traditionally known to manage anxiety and reduce agitation has been used to improve cognition in Alzheimer's patients, while sage and withania, two herbs with antioxidant, anti-inflammatory and memory enhancing qualities, also have the potential to benefit Alzheimer's sufferers.

While there is no magical recipe yet for defeating Alzheimer's disease, combining the remedies mentioned above together with those mentioned in the prevention section might provide Alzheimer's sufferers with some means for keeping this monstrous disorder at bay. Here is a list of the substances that can be taken on a daily basis. Testosterone might only be beneficial if levels are low.

- Oestradiol cream or troches 0.1-0.5mg for women
- Testosterone cream or troches 25-50mg for men
- Melatonin 3-9mg orally at night
- Vitamins B1, B2 and B3 100mg of each
- Vitamin B12 500mcg
- Folic acid 400mcg
- Vitamin C 1000mg
- Vitamin E 2000 i.u.
- Omega-3 fatty acids 2 grams

- Acetyl-L-carnitine 1 gram
- NADH 10mg
- Alpha-lipoic acid 200mg three times daily
- Coenzyme Q10 200mg
- Carnosine 1000mg
- Phosphatidylserine 200mg
- Curcumin 400mg
- Bacopa monniera (Brahmi) 100mg
- Vinca minor 80mg
- Ginkgo biloba 120mg
- Gotu kola 100mg
- Huperzine 100mcg
- Lemon balm 60 drops of standardised extract
- Sage 100mg
- Withania 100mg

PREVENTING AND TREATING PARKINSON'S DISEASE

After Alzheimer's disease Parkinson's is the second most common neurodegenerative disorder affecting approximately 1% of individuals over of the age of 60. Parkinson's disease attacks that part of the brain, which controls balance and movement, so that sufferers of this disorder experience increasing problems with walking and maintaining their sense of equilibrium, becoming increasingly stiff and rigid. To get around Parkinson's sufferers have to shuffle rather than move with any fluency and because they have difficulty moving their facial muscles they become increasingly expressionless with their emotions registering in a blank stare. Although the course of this disease can be rather protracted, like Alzheimer's this disorder is also progressive and unrelenting, leading to increasing incapacity.

We don't know yet what causes Parkinson's disease but it is thought to be related to a combination of genetic and environmental circumstances. Superimpose repeated environmental insults on genetic susceptibility and you will have the right combination that culminates in the development of Parkinson's disease. Regular exposure to pesticides and herbicides, the accumulation of metals such as mercury, lead, aluminium, copper, zinc and manganese, environmental toxins like MPTP (1-methyl, 4-phenyl, 1,2,3,6-tetrahydropyridine) used by drug addicts when injecting heroin, inflammation and excessive free radical stress are some of the key environmental elements that lead to Parkinson's disease. In some ways this is good news as all these factors are preventable.

Heavy metal overload, inflammation and free radical stress can be measured and treated appropriately. You might not be able to do much about your genes but you can have some impact on the kind of environment that affects the way your genes express themselves.

PREVENTING PARKINSON'S DISEASE

THE HORMONES

MELATONIN

Melatonin is the solitary hormone that has any capacity to put a stop to the build-up of free radicals that propel Parkinson's disease. There is an area of the brain called the substantia nigra where dopamine is produced and it is this chemical which governs motor behaviour. In an escalating fashion, free radicals gobble up the substantia nigra reducing its ability to provide the necessary dopamine that allows us to carry out our daily activities which then leads to all the deficits associated with Parkinson's. By restraining free radicals melatonin can contribute to the preservation of normal dopamine levels. What you can do is have your melatonin levels measured by salivary hormone assay performed just before you go to sleep and supplementing if your body is manufacturing insufficient melatonin.

VITAMINS, THE DIET and SPECIAL NUTRIENTS

In addition to optimising your melatonin levels employing a team of antioxidants would further buttress your defences against free radicals. Vitamins C, E, green tea and coenzyme Q10 would be the prime candidates for this role. One of the most important nutrients that protects the substantia nigra is the antioxidant glutathione and it is the depletion of this substance that makes this area of the brain so vulnerable to free radical attack. By increasing available glutathione you will be furnishing your brain with a vital nutrient that might be the major contributor to the prevention of Parkinson's disease. Because glutathione can be difficult to absorb when taken orally you can utilise N-acetylcysteine and alpha-lipoic acid both of which have the ability to provide you with sufficient amounts of glutathione. Consuming fruits and vegetables which are rich in antioxidants such as the berry fruits, apples, tomatoes, carrots and leafy green vegetables and limiting saturated fats, cooking oils and fried foods would also be highly beneficial. I was extremely surprised to discover that both caffeine and nicotine can prevent Parkinson's disease. For some reason Parkinson's disease is much more common in men and a recent study has revealed that those men who consume four cups or more of coffee a day have a lower incidence of this disorder. (64) Strangely, smokers also develop less Parkinson's disease. I don't think I have to remind you of the many dangers of cigarette smoking and drinking in excess of two cups of coffee a day. This would result in the loss of crucial nutrients such as magnesium and potassium as caffeine makes you urinate more often. Until modern science has discovered the reasons for the benefits of caffeine and nicotine I suggest that coffee lovers temper their enthusiasm for this beverage by not having more than two cups of coffee per day and stick to all the other means mentioned above for preventing Parkinson's disease.

Preventing Parkinson's disease
It would be wise to check your melatonin levels and only start taking this hormone if your levels are low.

- Melatonin 1-3mg at night
- Vitamin C 500mg daily
- Vitamin E 400mg of mixed tocopherols with 50mg of tocotrienols daily
- Green tea 2-4 cups daily
- Coenzyme Q10 100mg daily
- N-acetylcysteine 400mg daily
- Alpha-lipoic acid 200mg daily

TREATING PARKINSON'S DISEASE

MELATONIN

Melatonin stands alone as the only hormone which appears to have any say in the progression of Parkinson's disease. Unfortunately there are no studies showing that oestrogen, testosterone or DHEA are of any benefit.

VITAMINS, THE DIET AND SPECIAL NUTRIENTS

Large doses of coenzyme Q10 delay the evolution of Parkinson's disease. A German study has revealed that the administration of 360mg of coenzyme Q10 over a four-week period leads to a mild but significant improvement in symptoms. (65) Current thinking suggests that combining up to 2400mg per day of coenzyme Q10 with 1200i.u. of vitamin E might be the way forward. Vitamins C and D, alpha-lipoic acid, N-acetylcysteine, creatine, which is used to increase cellular energy, and the herbs ginseng and ginkgo biloba have all been shown in animal and cell culture studies to be beneficial for the management of Parkinson's disease principally by reducing free radical stress. One human trial has demonstrated that NADH, the energy booster, has a positive influence on Parkinson's disease.

An elegant Brazilian study has indicated that taking 30mg of riboflavin (vitamin B2) three times daily together with the elimination of red meat leads to significant improvements in the functional capabilities of Parkinson's patients. They were able to sleep better at night and enjoyed improved reasoning, higher motivation and reduced depression. (66.)

Increasing glutathione by utilising alpha-lipoic acid and N-acetylcysteine also helps to alleviate the symptoms of Parkinson's sufferers. An even more efficient way of delivering glutathione is via intravenous injection.

Dr Perlmutter of the 'Better Brain Book' fame has incorporated this approach at his clinic in the USA and has found that this leads to significant improvements in mobility, reduced tremor and better mood. To achieve these kinds of results this treatment needs to be administered three times weekly.

Omega-3 fatty acids, which reduce inflammation, may be of benefit while octacosanol, a substance found in wheat germ oil, was also found to reduce the symptoms of Parkinson's disease.

The most effective way to make meaningful inroads on all the debilitating features of Parkinson's disease is to adhere to a team approach when supplementing with hormones and nutrients.

This is the programme that can be utilised to manage Parkinson's disease.

- Melatonin 3-9mg at night
- Coenzyme Q10 600mg twice daily
- Vitamin E 600i.u. twice daily
- Vitamin C 500mg twice daily
- Vitamin D 1000 i.u. daily
- NADH 10mg daily
- Alpha-lipoic acid 200mg daily
- N-acetylcysteine 400mg twice daily
- Riboflavin 30mg three times daily
- Ginseng 200mg twice daily
- Ginkgo biloba 60mg twice daily
- Creatine 2 grams daily
- Omega-3 fatty acids found in fish oil 1 gram daily
- Octacosanol 5mg three times daily

CHAPTER 9

Walking the Tightrope That is the Immune System

As we age our immune systems become weaker and this makes us more vulnerable to infections and diseases like cancer. Paradoxically, components of our immune system, recognised as pro-inflammatory chemicals also known as cytokines such as interleukin-6 (IL-6) and tumour necrosis factor alpha (TNF alpha), also become more active which further increases our propensity to develop age-related diseases such as osteoporosis, Alzheimer's dementia and heart disease. Overproduction of IL-6 and TNF alpha have also been connected with lower muscle mass and weakness in older men and women and is thought to be associated with increasing frailty in the elderly. (1) (2)

While we need IL-6 and TNF alpha to mount an appropriate response to foreign invaders and to kill cancer cells, having excessive levels of these cytokines can be harmful and destructive. What we need to do is find the delicate balance that successfully ramps up our dwindling immune resources and simultaneously reduces the heat that IL-6 and TNF alpha are generating. This is how we can utilise hormones, vitamins and special nutrients to help achieve these objectives.

THE HORMONES
OESTROGEN

Oestrogen has a variety of benefits on the immune system. This hormone has the ability to increase B-cell and T-cell function, which comprise the two major arms of the immune system. Post-menopausal women on HRT were shown to have more B-cells, higher T-cell activity and generally enjoyed a reversal of the immune alterations associated with normal ageing. (3) Oestrogen also lessens the activity of IL-6 suggesting that pro-inflammatory damage can be minimised by the presence of this hormone. (4)

PROGESTERONE

Progesterone tones down the immune system making it more difficult for autoimmune diseases such as systemic lupus erythematosis (SLE) to establish themselves. Although for the most part having enough oestrogen is thought to benefit the immune system, in the case of SLE, oestrogen replacement could lead to flare-ups of this disease. In this scenario progesterone could be a useful moderator of oestrogen.

TESTOSTERONE

Testosterone's effects on immune function have not been widely investigated. This hormone is thought to be far less stimulating on the immune system than oestrogen. Men suffer less from autoimmune diseases such as SLE but at the same time have a reduced capacity to fight off viruses and parasitic infestations. On average women live ten to four years longer than men and this might have something to do with testosterone's waning ability to mobilise the immune system.

GROWTH HORMONE

Ageing witnesses a decline in the production of growth hormone and IGF-1, which coincides with the weakening of the immune system. Boosting growth hormone levels has been found to increase T-cells and B-cells as well as natural killer cells, which are powerful inhibitors of invading germs.

Another factor, which contributes to deterioration of the immune system, is the shrinking of the thymus gland located just above the breastbone, which has a major role in priming T-cells for action. Growth hormone has also been shown to regenerate the thymus gland, which restores T-cell function.

MELATONIN

Like growth hormone, melatonin has the ability to rejuvenate the thymus and stimulate the release of a number of immune-enhancing cells including immunoglobulins, CD4 cells, interferon and interleukin-2, which ward off viral infections. Melatonin also increases the production of thyroid hormones, which then enhance immune activity.

THYROID HORMONES

Thyroid hormones have a significant influence on the immune system. Although ageing is not associated with a profound reduction in thyroid hormone production there can be a significant diminution in the presence of these hormones which compromise immune function. Low levels of the thyroid hormone T3 lead to reduced activity of natural killer cells while supplementing with T3 increases the activity of these immune cells.

DEHYDROEPIANDROSTERONE (DHEA)
and CORTISOL

DHEA is also thought to be a potent promoter of the immune response. Cortisol has more suppressive and immunomodulatory effects. The secretion of cortisol remains stable with ageing while that of DHEA declines considerably, which possibly leads to the age-related loss in immune competence. DHEA has been demonstrated to neutralise the pro-inflammatory cytokine IL-6 while increasing interleukin-2 and natural killer cells, which makes it easier to combat invading micro-organisms. DHEA's effects on the immune system are remarkably similar to those of oestrogen and as DHEA is converted to this hormone it is possible that all the benefits of DHEA are due to this transformation.

It's not too difficult to notice that ageing, the deterioration of immune function and the lessening of hormone production occur concurrently. Bringing the immune system into balance by augmenting the production of these hormones might be the ideal way to fortify our body's defences against infections, cancers and degenerative diseases that intensify with ageing.

VITAMINS AND SPECIAL NUTRIENTS

If you're looking to support your immune system then vitamins A, B6, C, D and E together with zinc, selenium and coenzyme Q10 as well as the amino acids, L-arginine, glutathione and glycine are the nutrients that will provide you with the most assistance. Herbal remedies such as echinacea, garlic and andrographis in addition to resveratrol, green tea and curcumin will also help to boost your defences. Foods that have immune-enhancing properties include the flavonoids found in citrus fruits, blueberries, onions, apples and broccoli, the carotenoids in carrots, tomatoes and spinach and the phytosterols which reside in almonds, cashews, sesame and sunflower seeds.

TREATING HIV INFECTION

One of the most distressing experiences that I've had to negotiate in my 20 years of clinical practice was the day that I had to inform one of my male patients that he had HIV infection.   Although this event took place close to ten years ago that day is vividly etched in my memory. Mercifully, with the recent advances in medical treatments HIV infection no longer constitutes a death sentence and there are many HIV positive patients who are doing very well despite the presence of this virus. Nevertheless modern day treatments have their limitations and they are not without side effects. Therefore it is worthwhile evaluating the contribution that hormones, vitamins and special nutrients can make to the management of this condition.

GROWTH HORMONE

Despite the benefits of antiretroviral therapy, immune system depletion is still a problem during HIV infection. One of the most vital components of the immune system is natural killer cells as it is these cells that produce powerful antiviral agents such as interferon and tumour necrosis factor which target viral replication in the early stages of viral infection. Unfortunately natural killer cells often find themselves significantly compromised with HIV disease, which makes it that much easier for the virus to gain a foothold in the body. Notwithstanding the advantages of antiretroviral therapy, this form of treatment can have adverse effects on natural killer cells, which does limit their capacity to effectively target the HIV virus.

Help may be at hand in the form of growth hormone therapy. A clinical trial completed in the United Kingdom has demonstrated that growth hormone injections were able to improve natural killer cell numbers and function. This allowed these cells to produce more interferon, which helped them to engage the virus more effectively. (5) Another study conducted in the USA has further detailed the immune-boosting benefits of growth hormone injections showing that this treatment has the power to increase the size of the thymus which undoubtably enhances immune system capabilities as evidenced by the increase in CD4 cells. (6) CD4 cells are specialized white blood cells that direct other cells to fight an infection caused by germs, like HIV.

HIV infection can also lead to a significant loss of muscle mass with antiretroviral therapy resulting in the accumulation of fat around the midriff, which is associated with insulin resistance and the elevation of cholesterol levels. Growth hormone treatment can reverse these deleterious trends by improving lean muscle tissue, reducing the build-up of fat that surrounds the trunk and elevating HDL cholesterol levels. The nervous system is another repository for the ubiquitous HIV virus where it can wreak endless havoc and devastation. This can culminate in the development of cognitive impairment and even sometimes dementia. Growth hormone, with its neuroprotective and nerve growth promoting effects, has been shown to improve cognitive function in HIV sufferers with impaired mental capacity, suggesting that this treatment might be an effective means for withstanding the damage which this virus can inflict on the brain. (7)

Another adverse consequence of antiretroviral therapy is the harm that this medication can inflict on the mitochondria, the battery of the cell, leading to diminished energy production and fatigue. Growth hormone treatment can reduce this side effect by helping the cell to utilise oxygen more efficiently in order to generate energy.

If growth hormone levels are low this form of treatment offers a wide range of benefits for HIV sufferers.

TESTOSTERONE

If testosterone levels are low supplementing with this hormone can also help rebuild lost muscle mass while at the same time improving muscle strength and boosting mood. Combining this form of therapy with exercise and weight training can lead to even greater gains in muscle performance. For HIV positive women with low testosterone levels who suffer from loss of muscle tissue and fatigue, treatment with this hormone might also be an effective means for overturning this trend.

DHEA

There aren't many studies which have explored the gains that can be achieved by taking DHEA. However there is a connection between the HIV-associated lipodystrophy syndrome alluded to in the above segment, which is associated with the massing of fat around the tummy, raised cholesterol levels and insulin resistance, with low DHEA and elevated cortisol. Although there haven't been any clinical trials which investigated whether DHEA could alter this metabolic profile there is evidence that the absence of these abnormalities are associated with raised DHEA levels suggesting that this hormone might exert a positive influence on this condition. Remember that DHEA can improve mental function and boost the immune system in a number of ways.

OESTROGEN

One of the added problems that HIV positive women have to face is the increased possibility of developing a heart attack due to occluded arteries. Oestrogen has the potential to prevent this development by blocking the inflammatory cells which initiate this process. For those women with low oestrogen, taking this hormone might provide added protection against heart disease.

MELATONIN

There is some, albeit limited, evidence that melatonin has the ability to boost CD4 cell counts and improve the prognosis of HIV positive patients.

THYROID HORMONES

Deficiencies of thyroid hormones may be common amongst HIV sufferers and as these hormones have the ability to stimulate the immune system integrating this treatment might be extremely helpful.

Managing HIV infection
Hormones might only be helpful if levels are low and should be monitored periodically by means of blood tests.

- Growth hormone ¼-1 i.u. by injection daily
- Testosterone cream or troches 25-50mg for men
- Testosterone cream or troches 1mg topically for women

- DHEA 25mg orally for men
- DHEA 10-25 mg orally for women
- Oestradiol cream or troches ½ - 2mg for women
- Melatonin 3-9mg at night
- Thyroid hormones 22.4mcg T4 and 6.8mcg T3 daily

THE VITAMINS

At the end of 2003 approximately 40 million people were infected with the HIV virus worldwide. The real tragedy is the extent to which the virus has ravaged vast segments of the population in sub-Saharan Africa, which at conservative estimates amounts to around 70% of the total number of persons with HIV/AIDS. What is worse is that in this part of the world malnutrition is rife which makes it that much more difficult to fight HIV infection. Low levels of vitamins A, B complex, C and E are the norm for these people and this has been associated with disease progression.

In 1995 over one thousand HIV-infected pregnant women in Dar-es-Salaam, Tanzania, were provided with vitamin supplements including 20mg of vitamin B1, 20mg of vitamin B2, 25mg of vitamin B6, 100mg of niacin, 50micrograms of vitamin B12, 500mg of vitamin C, 30mg of vitamin E and 0.8mg of folic acid. These women were monitored until the end of the study in 2003. (8) The results of this extended trial were extremely encouraging. Significantly fewer of these women developed full-blown AIDS or died compared with a placebo group who didn't receive this vitamin regimen. CD4 and CD8 counts also improved considerably and viral loads were lower. These positive findings were replicated by another experiment in Toronto, Canada, which revealed that three months of treatment with vitamin E comprising 800 i.u. of DL-alpha-tocopherol acetate combined with 1000mg of vitamin C reduced viral load and free radical status. (9)

Other studies conducted in Poland and France have also demonstrated that supplementing with vitamins, A, C and E together with other antioxidants including beta-carotene, N-acetylcysteine, selenium and gingko biloba protected DNA from free radical damage, improved mitochondrial function and elevated CD4 counts, indicating a stimulating effect on the immune system. (10) (11) Animal trials have shown benefits with vitamin E, while supplementing with the B vitamin complex and especially vitamin B12, has resulted in improved natural killer cell activity and was even able to reverse a case of advanced AIDS dementia complex. (12)

My advice for those with HIV infection is to supplement with the full range of vitamins. Here is the list together with suggested doses:

- Beta-carotene 20mg daily
- Vitamin B complex 2 daily comprised of 100mg of each B vitamin together with 250micrograms of vitamin B12 and folic acid
- Vitamin C 500mg twice daily
- Vitamin E 400i.u. made up of a mixed tocopherols plus 50mg of the tocotrienols

ANTIOXIDANTS, SPECIAL NUTRIENTS, HERBAL MEDICINES and OTHER NUTRIENTS

Selenium is intimately connected with the body's antioxidant defence mechanism and vitally important for the immune system. T-cells are activated and natural killer cells are stimulated by the presence of selenium. Selenium prevents the HIV virus from multiplying and boosting selenium levels has been shown to substantially reduce the risk of mortality in HIV infected persons. (13) (14) Conversely, worsening of HIV infection, which coincides with a progressive loss of CD4 protection, runs hand in glove with declining selenium levels. Selenium deficiency contributes significantly to increasing HIV mortality on a worldwide basis. Even if the diet contains selenium, which is found in fish, eggs, Brazil nuts, cashews, garlic, wholegrain cereals and alfalfa, supplementing with extra selenium would provide the immune system with much needed fortification.

The research results with zinc are less consistent. Most studies do show an improvement in CD4 counts and immune function with zinc supplementation. However, there is one American study which found that dietary zinc intake was associated with an apparent increase in the rate of progression and mortality due to HIV infection. (15) It's probably best not to supplement with more than 30mg of elemental zinc daily. If you want to be totally safe, monitoring zinc status via a zinc taste test would be advisable. Only supplementing if your taste buds don't respond positively to that furry zinc taste, which indicates a zinc deficiency, would be advisable.

One of the most important antioxidants and immune balancing agents is glutathione. It's not that easy to absorb glutathione when this nutrient is taken orally but it is possible to encourage the body to manufacture extra amounts of glutathione by supplementing with N-acetylcysteine and alpha-lipoic acid.   Replenishing glutathione has been shown to decrease HIV replication, preserve CD4 cell counts and to lead to a considerably greater chance of survival over a two-year period in a group of HIV positive men who were taking N-acetylcysteine.

The amino acid L-glutamine has been used to rebuild lost muscle tissue. Acetyl-L-carnitine, which helps with the metabolism of fat to provide energy, has the ability to protect cells from the side effects of AZT therapy (an anti-HIV medication also known as Retrovir) while providing the added bonus of increasing CD4 counts. The antioxidant coenzyme Q10 has also been demonstrated to boost CD4 counts.

Maitake MD-fraction, a Japanese mushroom extract, has the ability to increase helper T-cells and to inhibit the HIV virus. Phytosterols, a plant compound with immune-enhancing properties, has been administered in a clinical trial in South Africa with evidence that this compound was able to increase helper T-cells and reduce the viral load in a group of HIV positive patients. (16)

There is preliminary evidence that giving beta glucans, a compound found in oats and barley, by means of intravenous injections can increase levels of CD4 cells and reduce viral replication.

Whey protein, which increases glutathione, also has the ability to reverse weight loss.

There is some evidence that the herbs echinacea, curcumin, andrographis, astragalus, green tea and an extract of liquorice called stronger neo-minophagen C can strengthen the immune system by increasing natural killer cells and CD4 counts which helps to reduce viral levels.

> **Here is a summary of all the natural remedies that play a role in heightening the immune response, which helps to confront the HIV virus:**
>
> - Selenium 200micrograms daily
> - Zinc 30mg daily
> - N-acetylcysteine 600mg twice daily
> - Alpha-lipoic acid 200mg daily
> - L-glutamine 40grams daily
> - Acetyl-L-carnitine 1500mg twice daily
> - Maitake MD-fraction 35-70mls daily
> - Phytosterols 20mg daily
> - Beta glucans 110mg intravenously twice weekly
> - Whey protein 20grams daily
> - Echinacea 100mg twice daily
> - Curcumin 400mg daily
> - Andrographis 100mg daily
> - Astragalus 2 grams daily
> - Green tea 2-4 cups daily
> - Stronger neo-minophagen C 100-200mls intravenously twice weekly

Just a brief postscript to this section - there is a publication entitled 'The Immune Restoration Handbook' found at www.keephope.net in which the American author Mark Konlee cites a number of remedies that boost natural killer cell production including 4-life transfer factor, low dose naltrexone, inositol hexaphosphate and garlic. He also documents a vast array of other treatments such as coconut milk, essiac tea, the herbs black walnut, olive leaf extract and wormwood, an African herbal formulation called 'impi' and a Chinese herbal compound known as 'revivo', which have been used to treat HIV infection.

Some of the testimonials presented in the book to support these therapies are highly impressive but the evidence for most of these is anecdotal and not based on clinical trials. The website www.lowdosenaltrexone.org provides further information about the use of naltrexone to treat the HIV virus.

TREATING MULTIPLE SCLEROSIS

If HIV infection constitutes a challenge in dealing with a fragile immune system, multiple sclerosis demands that we find ways to modulate an immune response that seems to have become overactive. Although the precise cause of multiple sclerosis has yet to be determined, it is thought that this disease may be driven at least in part by an autoimmune process suggesting that the body's immune system has become overzealous by inadvertently attacking its own nervous system.

Early adulthood is the usual time when this disease strikes with numbness, impaired vision, loss of balance, weakness and altered psychological states being common symptoms. These symptoms can come and go with the manifestation of this disorder often fluctuating over extended periods of time sometimes for up to 30years. However in some unfortunate cases severe disability can be the outcome.

Multiple sclerosis is far more common in women and the precise reason for this is rather complex and still somewhat unclear but here's the intriguing part - both female and male hormones might offer a plausible option for treating multiple sclerosis.

OESTROGEN

Multiple sclerosis has been noted to improve during pregnancy. This is a time when excessive amounts of oestrogen in the form of oestradiol, as well as oestriol and progesterone are manufactured. Oestriol is the female hormone that is mostly produced during pregnancy, and it is this hormone which has been found in clinical trials to lead to discernible clinical benefits.

A group of women who were given 8mg of oestriol orally per day for six months experienced favourable changes in their immune systems and reduced numbers of lesions in their nervous systems indicating that part of the damage inflicted as a result of this disease was being repaired. Their mental function also improved. (17) This is a highly encouraging outcome. The same research team has proposed that low doses of oestradiol, the stronger oestrogen, might also be useful for managing multiple sclerosis.

However it's not only women that might benefit from the therapeutic effects of oestriol and oestradiol. This form of treatment might equally be applicable for men. Male mice with a disease similar to multiple sclerosis have been shown to respond positively to oestriol. (18) Although this has yet to find its way into a clinical trial on men, the possibility now exists that oestriol can be used to treat both women and men who suffer from multiple sclerosis. The appropriate dosage of oestriol for men has yet to be determined. Our bodies have each other's hormones albeit in lesser amounts and these operate in weird and wonderful ways to impact upon our health. Amazingly, it appears that there are more ways than we could have imagined for using these powerful chemicals to treat those diseases that impact on our wellness.

TESTOSTERONE

Those men who balk at using oestriol can rest easy. Taking testosterone might offer another therapeutic alternative for the management of multiple sclerosis. Men with low testosterone levels are more vulnerable to developing this disease. In male mice testosterone has protective advantages and the same male mice, when administered dihydrotestosterone, the more potent form of this hormone, experienced improvements in a disease that is similar to multiple sclerosis. (19)

DEHYDROEPIANDROSTERONE (DHEA)

In laboratory animals DHEA has been shown to have potent anti-inflammatory properties and to decrease the damage to the nervous system associated with multiple sclerosis. This has yet to be replicated in humans but it does suggest that DHEA may prove a viable proposition for managing multiple sclerosis.

THYROID HORMONES

One of the problems associated with multiple sclerosis is the progressive destruction of the lining that surrounds the nerves called the myelin sheaths. Even with conventional treatment this process, which is known as demyelination, can lead to the increasing disability associated with this disease. The application of thyroid hormone might resolve this dilemma. In rats thyroid hormone has been shown to promote the growth of myelin sheaths in those animals suffering from a multiple sclerosis like disease, which leads to the restoration of normal nervous tissue. (20)

Thyroid hormone might yet prove to be a highly useful means for repairing the damaged nervous system that lies at the core of multiple sclerosis.

Before commencing any form of hormone therapy it would be advisable to have your hormone levels measured. Although all the animal experimentation doesn't clarify this issue, making use of hormones might only be appropriate if your levels are low. Oestriol can be evaluated in both sexes via salivary hormone assays.

Hormone treatments for multiple sclerosis:

- Oestriol 8mg orally daily for women or
- Oestradiol cream ¼ -2mg daily
- Testosterone cream or troches 30-50mg for men
- DHEA cream or orally 25mg daily for men
- DHEA cream or orally 15-25mg daily for women
- Thyroid hormones in the form of compounded physiologic thyroid T4=22.4mcg and T3=6.8mcg

THE VITAMINS

The incidence of multiple sclerosis is higher in areas where there is less exposure to sunlight, which diminishes the potentially protective benefits of vitamin D. In mice with a disease resembling multiple sclerosis, the administration of vitamin D has been shown to reduce disease activity. There are precious few clinical trials which have investigated the benefits of vitamin D in multiple sclerosis patients, however one conducted in 1986 did demonstrate that combining 5000i.u. of vitamin D with calcium (16mg/kg/day) and magnesium (10mg/kg/day) limited flare-ups of this disease by 59%. (21)

Vitamin B12 is necessary for the formation of myelin. This time both animal and human trials indicate that vitamin B12 can lead to clinical improvements and a lessening of disability in patients with multiple sclerosis. (22)

You can supplement with vitamin B12 orally but to achieve a more powerful effect injecting with this vitamin would be more useful. The oral dose of vitamin B12 would be 250mcg twice daily whereas with injections, 20mg of methylcobalamin injected weekly, the form of vitamin B12 that is best delivered to the nervous system where it is needed, would be a good initial dose.

Retinoic acid, a vitamin A derivative, has been demonstrated to be of benefit in the same animal model of multiple sclerosis that has been alluded to all along in this section. Retinoic acid has similar benefits to vitamin D in modulating the immune system, which combats the destructive effects that this disease has on the nervous system. Retinoic acid is available on special prescription.

There is the notion that the accumulation of free radicals, if not being a primary cause of multiple sclerosis, at least contributes to worsening of this disease. Although there is limited evidence, supplementing with vitamin C and E might help to curb repeated attacks of this disorder.

Vitamin supplements for the management of multiple sclerosis:

- Vitamin D 5000i.u. daily
- Vitamin B12 250mcg twice daily
- Retinoic acid 20mg daily
- Vitamin C 500mg twice daily
- Vitamin E 400i.u comprising mixed tocopherols and 50mg mixed tocotrienols daily

---

ANTIOXIDANTS AND SPECIAL NUTRIENTS

Alpha-lipoic acid is another impressive performer against the animal form of multiple sclerosis suggesting that this nutrient may also have a role to play in the management of multiple sclerosis. (23) One of the ways to attack this disease is to reduce inflammation by restricting your consumption of the kinds of foods that are thought to increase this process including margarines, vegetable oils, red meat and dairy products, as well as by taking supplements of fish or flaxseed oils. One trial has supported this, revealing that the combination of omega-3 fatty acids found in fish oil with vitamins was able to cut back on exacerbations of this disease. (24)

Another nutrient that has intriguing benefits with regard to multiple sclerosis is histamine. This nutrient is purported to stimulate regrowth of myelin around nerves, which has the potential to reverse all the damage that is characteristic of multiple sclerosis. Histamine when applied to the skin has been found to improve a number of symptoms including balance control, fatigue and cognitive function.

Acetyl-L-carnitine, which helps with the generation of

energy, has also been found to ameliorate fatigue associated with multiple sclerosis. Magnesium, the perennial nervous system stabilizer, has also been shown to have a positive impact on multiple sclerosis by reducing relapse rates.

Supplementary treatment for multiple sclerosis:

- Alpha-lipoic acid 200mg daily
- Fish oil 2 grams daily
- Histamine cream 3-6grms daily
- Acetyl-L-carnitine 1gram twice daily
- Magnesium 400mg twice daily

As part of your treatment programme it is also important that you have the appropriate blood tests, which evaluate your candida status via your antibody levels, and gluten intolerance by means of gliadin antibodies. If these are present it would be extremely helpful to treat these according to the protocol outlined in chapter three.

If you have mercury fillings having these removed might also be beneficial.

Beyond Botox & Propecia: Combatting Wrinkles & Hair Loss

COMBATTING WRINKLES & HAIR LOSS

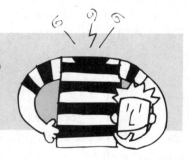

'That's one way to stop looking your age'

One of the nicest compliments we can receive is to hear that most cherished affirmation, 'you don't look your age.' It's the kind of flattery we all yearn for. We live in a culture that worships youthfulness and I don't think I'm giving away any major secrets here by affirming that everyone we meet will have a go at guessing our age by the status of our skin with our facial features receiving the most critical scrutiny. As I'm an anti-ageing doctor and part of the health and wellness industry I'm subject to this kind of evaluation all the time. Due to the misguided pursuits of my youth when I was an avid sun worshipper I have all the telltale signs of what is scientifically described as photoageing.

To put it simply I have wrinkles clearly etched around my

eyes and forehead which makes my struggle to look younger than my years an uphill one, and I'm not about to submit to the visible benefits of botox. As it turns out there is a lot that can be done in the form of hormonal therapies, vitamin, herbal and antioxidant treatments, which are mostly applied topically, as well as dietary changes to impact the ravages of time and sun on our skin.

The same factors that promote ageing in the rest of your body also target your skin. Free radical stress, inflammation and poor sugar metabolism are thought to be the primary causes of skin ageing and wrinkles. This means that if you can neutralise these processes you can at least have some chance of preserving a youthful appearance. Even the damaging effects of ultraviolet radiation, which result from overexposure to the sun's rays, are primarily due to the generation of free radicals. This would imply that using antioxidants, which inhibit free radicals, might be able to limit the harmful effects of the sun.

Just to recap - excess free radical stress results from deep fried foods, packaged biscuits and cakes, preservatives, pesticides and herbicides in foods, pollution and passive smoking to name some of the major contributors to this potentially destructive process. Inflammation can result from abnormal germs in the bowel including candida overgrowth as well as food allergy. I consult with many patients who present with skin conditions including dermatitis, psoriasis, acne and other debilitating skin conditions. Time and again I find that candida infestations and food allergy especially gluten intolerance are associated with their problems. Treating these often leads to significant improvements and if you are going to look after the health of your skin then you need to identify these underlying processes and eliminate them in the appropriate fashion.

Imperfect sugar metabolism can also lead to inflammation. This results from the consumption of foods with a high glycaemic index such as white bread, white rice, potato, sweet biscuits, cereals like corn flakes and sultana bran, dried fruit, bananas, mangoes, pineapple and melons. These foods lead to a rapid build-up of sugar in your bloodstream, which coats the protein in your tissues. This can also happen in your skin where the combination of sugar and collagen weakens the elasticity of your skin leading to the formation of deep wrinkles. It is far healthier to consume foods with a low glycaemic index, which leads to blood sugar levels that are steady and stable over time and more nourishing of your skin. These include green vegetables, all fruits except those mentioned, basmati rice, spaghetti, buckwheat pasta, soybeans, baked beans and lentils.

Your skin also thrives on a healthy supply of fats and protein. There are good fats and fats that are harmful. The good fats are found in avocado, fresh raw nuts like cashews, walnuts, almonds and macadamias, flaxseed, extra virgin olive oil and the small fish that have low levels of mercury such as sardines, herring, salmon and mackerel, while the bad fats comprise margarines, vegetable oils including corn oil, safflower oil and canola oil as well as beef, veal, pork and lamb.

You can get the protein you need from beans combined with corn, nuts or rice, lentils, eggs, the fish I've just mentioned and if you're going to have meat, turkey and chicken (the free range option would be preferable) in addition to which lean red meat eaten two to three times a week would do just nicely. Vegetarians often have a problem getting sufficient amounts of protein and I always advise those who don't include meat or fish in their diet to take supplementary protein in the form of rice and whey powder. The delicious smoothie I've already mentioned combines these two with rice milk and yoghurt. This provides around 30-40 grams of protein, which is more than half of your daily protein requirements.

Adequate hydration is also important for your skin, and while the scientists are still squabbling over the exact amount that we all need, it would be a good idea to drink 4-6 glasses daily. As you have to be reasonably dehydrated before you start becoming thirsty you can't really use thirst to assess your water needs, and it's best just to get into some form of routine whereby you're making sure that you obtain the amount of hydration that serves the needs of your skin.

Once you're on the healthy diet we can explore the ways by which hormones, vitamins, antioxidants and other special nutrients can help you to prevent skin ageing.

THE HORMONES

OESTROGEN

If you're currently going through menopause then you may be noticing to your dismay that your skin is becoming increasingly dry and losing its firmness, suppleness and elasticity. Sadly this is going to lead to a progressive deepening of your facial creases and that dreaded telltale sign of ageing, wrinkling. This is principally caused by a reduction in collagen, tissue hyaluronic acid and glycoaminglycans which are substances in the underlying skin tissue that are primarily responsible for looking after skin hydration and preserving healthy, youthful skin. These are the signs which we're all so desperately trying to avoid, and if we can't avert the effects of ageing there's always botox or the surgeon's scalpel.

You might not have to resort to these wonders of modern medicine. Oestrogen has the ability to prevent and even reverse all these distressing features of skin ageing. This hormone has been shown to maintain and increase skin thickness by increasing the collagen, glycoaminglycans and hyaluronic acid content of your skin tissue, which also preserves hydration and elasticity. (1) What this does is to preserve skin suppleness and prevent slackness from occurring. Hormone replacement therapy in the form of either Premarin, oestriol or oestradiol applied to the skin has been found to decrease small wrinkles and to reduce wrinkle depth. Studies have also demonstrated that postmenopausal women on hormone replacement therapy have fewer wrinkles and a significantly higher collagen content than untreated women. (2) Oestrogen also improves the blood supply to the skin and makes it easier for wounds to heal.

How can you enjoy the benefits of oestrogen? I have indicated all along in this book that I view hormone treatment as a long-term strategy to limit the effects of ageing so my first suggestion is to have your hormone levels measured and this would include both oestradiol and oestriol. To measure oestriol you might have to use the salivary method, as blood tests are not freely available. You can then apply these hormones topically to your wrinkles either in the form of 0.3% oestriol or 0.01% oestradiol cream. The changes can be subtle which means that you might only notice improvements after 2-3 months.

It would also be prudent to have your hormone levels monitored when you're on such a programme as I do with all my patients to ensure that these are maintained within a healthy range. My advice is not to view your skin in isolation but to incorporate the management of your body's largest organ (yes it is your skin) in a holistic health programme, which includes an evaluation of all your other organ systems. This way any benefits that oestrogen treatment might have for your skin can be assessed along with all the other advantages this hormone might offer.

DHEA has anti-inflammatory and antioxidant potential as well as the ability to protect skin and blood vessels in the face of burn injuries. Melatonin also protects against sunburn and testosterone increases skin thickness in women and possibly also in men. Thyroid hormone deficiency contributes to dry, flaky skin, which suggests that optimising thyroid hormone levels would be beneficial for your skin. Although clinical trials haven't yet demonstrated that these hormones have the ability to reduce wrinkling these powerful chemicals have some promise in the fight to stave off the external effects of ageing.

THE VITAMINS

VITAMIN A

The topical form of vitamin A, which is available on prescription, is called Retin-A (tretinoin) and this has been documented in placebo-controlled trials to reduce wrinkling. (3) What you have to do is apply this cream in very small amounts to your skin at night as this treatment can cause some inflammation and redness, which is unsightly. Over-the-counter products, which incorporate vitamin A in the form of retinol and retinyl palmitate, might reduce shallow wrinkling but because these creams are far weaker than the prescription product the effects are less dramatic and can be less satisfying.

VITAMIN C

Vitamin C has the ability to stimulate collagen production and to reduce the effects of long-term sun damage. One clinical trial conducted over a six-month period demonstrated that the application of 5% vitamin C cream resulted in a significant reduction in small and coarse wrinkles as well as an improvement in firmness, smoothness and hydration. (4) Cellex-C, another form of topical vitamin C, has also been shown over a three-month period to lead to substantial improvements in an assessment of skin roughness, laxity and wrinkling. (5)

VITAMIN E

Vitamin E is a fat or lipid-soluble antioxidant, which makes it a vitally important nutrient for protecting cell membranes and the skin, which is lipid-rich. The problem that has often beset clinical trials is delivering vitamin E to the skin in a form which can be activated. One trial which compared the application of a topical cream consisting of 5% vitamin E to one side of the face with a placebo to the other did establish the superiority of this treatment for reducing length of facial lines and depth of wrinkles. (6) Numerous animal studies have shown that vitamin E has the ability to prevent sun-induced skin damage and to protect against the development of skin cancer. Interestingly the combination of vitamins C, E and melatonin was able to protect human skin from the damaging effects of ultraviolet radiation. Most experts agree however, that homing in on an effective form of vitamin E cream can be a tricky affair.

Nicotinamide, which is one of the two principal forms of the B-complex vitamin niacin or vitamin B3, has been shown to have some usefulness in preventing skin ageing by preventing water loss and increasing fatty tissue under the skin when this vitamin was administered in the form of a 4%gel.

ANTIOXIDANTS, HERBAL REMEDIES AND SPECIAL NUTRIENTS

Alpha-lipoic acid with its unique antioxidant and anti-inflammatory properties and its ability to recycle other antioxidants such as vitamins C and E has also been shown to have a positive impact on facial wrinkling by reducing vertical lines on the upper lip and fine lines around the eyes. Alpha-lipoic acid can also convert vitamin A to retinoic acid, a more potent form of this vitamin, and in another trial the application of 5% alpha-lipoic acid cream to the face for 12 weeks was able to decrease pigmentation, puffiness under the eyes, fine lines and skin roughness. Almost 80% of the subjects included in this trial noticed tangible improvements with this therapy. (7)

As is the case with the other vitamins the levels of coenzyme Q10 in the skin also diminish with ageing and, although the clinical trials investigating the benefits of this nutrient are sparse, there is evidence that skin cells pre-treated with coenzyme Q10 had less UVA-induced (ultraviolet light with type A rays) oxidative damage compared with controls. Another trial on 20 elderly volunteers revealed that the application of this nutrient around the eye lead to a 27% reduction in wrinkle depth compared with a control cream administered around the other eye. (8)

Soy is another nutrient that is gaining popularity in anti-ageing preparations due to its weak oestrogen-like effects. Soybean extracts have DNA-protective benefits, antipigmentary capabilities and can boost hyaluronic acid in the skin, which makes this nutrient an attractive proposition for managing the skin changes that occur over time.

Dr Nicholas Perricone, an American dermatologist who has written extensively on the natural management of skin ageing including a book called 'The Perricone Prescription,' which is a very worthwhile read, is very impressed with a substance called dimethylaminoethanol or DMAE, in short touted as the next best thing to help firm sagging skin especially around the face and neck. There is one trial which shows that a gel containing 3% DMAE goes some way to improving skin firmness. (9)

Skin peels with alpha-Hydroxyacids (AHAs) are commonly used to remove the superficial layers of the skin and replace these with more youthful cells. A variety of strengths of AHAs have been used ranging from 20-70%. Recent evidence indicates that polyhydroxy acids can achieve similar results to AHAs at a lower potency and with less stinging and burning, suggesting that this treatment might be a better option.

Rejuvenex cream developed by the Life Extension Foundation in the USA, which you will find described at www.lef.org, contains a number of the natural substances that I've described in the above segment including glycolic acid, purported to be the most potent of the AHAs. If you desire the full benefits of a skin peel with AHAs you should consult with a physician such as a dermatologist or a plastic surgeon who is familiar with the application of this treatment.

I have used Rejuvenex together with just about all the creams that contain all these substances and I would have to say that the results are subtle, probably because I have deep wrinkles. If you have fine lines and rather superficial wrinkles then you may be pleasantly surprised with the positive benefits of these topical agents over time. Hormonal applications of oestrogen, if appropriate, might also be highly useful but if you have my type of skin and you are expecting a facelift you might be setting yourself up for disappointment.

You should have your hormone levels measured before you utilise this therapy.

- Oestriol 0.3%
- Oestradiol 0.01%
- Retin-A 0.05%
- Vitamin C 5%
- Cellex-C
- Vitamin E 5%
- Nicotinamide gel 4%
- Alpha-lipoic acid 5%
- DMAE 3%

BATTLING HAIR LOSS

' Oh what I'd do for a full head of hair'

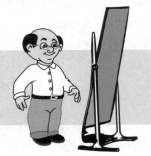

Another disturbing sign of ageing is hair loss. It's an event that both sexes have to deal with, as they get older. Among men and women hair growth flourishes between the ages of 15-30, starts to slow down from age 40-50 and is increasingly lost from the age of 50. A survey conducted in America in 2003 indicates that in that country 19.5 million women lose hair in some form compared with 33 million men. (10) Male-pattern baldness starts at the temples and also includes the top of the head. Female-pattern baldness causes the hair to thin out all over.   Stress, gluten intolerance, deficiencies of essential nutrients including iron, the B vitamin group, folic acid, selenium, and copper as well as hormonal imbalance are contributing factors to this scourge of ageing. Simple blood tests will identify excessive stress levels, nutrient deficiencies and hormonal imbalance while a hair mineral analysis can assess selenium and copper status. Conventional treatments for men include minoxidil, a topical lotion applied to the scalp, and finasteride or propecia, a tablet, which decreases dihydrotestosterone, the stronger male hormone, thought to be one of the primary instigators of hair loss in men and possibly also in women.

Although the shaven look is becoming more popular there are still a large number of men, myself included, who are engaged in the battle to preserve as much hair as possible. For women this is a no-brainer.   Aside from a few celebrities opting for a reduced mane of flowing locks, parting with their hair is not desired by most of the women I know. Aside from medical therapies, exploring hormonal status and using natural alternatives do offer other options for treatment.

THE HORMONES

As women approach menopause testosterone levels go into minor decline while oestrogen and sometimes thyroid hormone levels can diminish quite precipitously.   For those women who suffer from hair loss, fatigue, insomnia and depression it would be pertinent to have your oestrogen and thyroid hormone levels measured especially thyroxine or T4. If these are low, re-establishing normal levels of these hormones with oestradiol and thyroid hormone treatment might be able to reverse many of these alarming symptoms including hair loss. I have seen this many times in my practice and the truth is you don't have to resort to medications like anti-depressants, sleeping tablets, or pharmaceuticals that treat hair loss, to manage these problems. Oestradiol can be applied to the scalp to treat hair loss in women and even in men for that matter. This has been done in Europe for some time now with gratifying results. 17 alpha-oestradiol, a weakened form of the female hormone 17 beta-oestradiol, which is the oestradiol to which I've been referring in this book, has been found to be an effective treatment when used by men. (11) This form of hormonal treatment seems to work by reducing the effects of dihydrotestosterone. Women with hair loss can have their oestrogen levels measured before commencing such treatment while men can use this new form of oestrogen (called 17 alpha-oestradiol) to treat their receding hairlines.

Another fascinating trial has demonstrated that the combination of growth hormone, thyroid hormone, in the form of thyroxine, and insulin applied in a gel to the scalp of a group of men stopped hair loss and caused new hair growth which was highly effective. While the authors don't go into the reasons for the effectiveness of this treatment the success of this therapy, which was also side-effect free, makes this unique formulation a highly attractive proposition for restoring hair growth. (12)

THE SPECIAL NUTRIENTS

Saw palmetto is the herb used to treat enlargement of the prostate. It does this by lowering dihydrotestosterone, the same hormone associated with hair loss. It didn't take research scientists long to cotton on to the idea that this herb might also be effective for treating hair loss. This is exactly what has been demonstrated. Saw palmetto 200mg, combined with other natural remedies including beta-sitosterol 50mg, lecithin 50mg, inositol 100mg, phosphatidylcholine 25mg, niacin 15mg and biotin 100micrograms, was able to reduce the area of a bald spot and to stimulate hair growth over a four-month period. (13)

Ketaconazole is an anti-fungal medication, which has been used in shampoos to treat dandruff. It has also been discovered that ketaconazole has the ability to inhibit dihydrotestosterone and the long-term use of shampoos containing 2% ketaconazole used 2-4 times per week for 21 weeks was able to promote hair growth in a group of men between the ages of 21-33. (14)

Aside from making sure that you're getting enough iron, zinc, selenium and B vitamins you need to consume sufficient amounts of protein. Supplementary amino acids, the building blocks of protein, including L-lysine, L-cystine, L-methionine and L-cysteine, might be beneficial along with sulphur-rich foods including cabbage, eggs and garlic. Procyanidin B-2 is an antioxidant compound found in apples that has shown in a placebo-controlled study to promote significant hair regrowth when applied twice daily to the scalp in the form of a topical treatment over a four-month period. (15) This doesn't mean that eating lots of apples will do the trick as you will probably need to get hold of this specific compound and apply it to you scalp as per the protocol in this study.

To give you the final verdict on the success of these treatments I have used most of them and I have found that my hair loss has ceased and on a good hair day it certainly appears to me that regrowth is happening. My suggestion is to try these remedies for a 4-6 month period and see if there are any benefits.

Before you commence any hormonal treatment I recommend once again that you have your hormones measured.

Natural remedies for managing hair loss:

- T4=22.4mcg sustained release compounded physiologic thyroid taken daily
  T3=6.8mcg sustained release compounded physiologic thyroid taken daily
- Oestradiol for women 0.1% applied to scalp daily
- Ketaconazole 2% applied to scalp 4 times per week
- Procyanidin 1% applied to scalp twice daily
- Saw palmetto 200mg orally daily
- Beta-sitosterol 50mg orally daily
- Lecithin 50mg orally daily
- Inositol 100mg orally daily
- Phosphatidylcholine 25mg daily
- Niacin 15mg daily
- Biotin 100micrograms daily

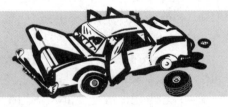

Have a check-up
before it's to late

It would be a wonderful world if everyone were on a wellness or anti-ageing programme. If we all took better care of ourselves before we became unwell then the world would be in much better shape. Here's your chance to be smart and get in early before it's too late. If you're constantly feeling unwell and fatigued, your memory and sex drive are rapidly dwindling and you've put on a truckload of weight then you'd be really wise to sit up and pay attention.

These are the signs that your body is ageing prematurely. This is a clear indication that your hormones and vitamins aren't doing their job and that your cells are giving you very unambiguous signs that they are struggling. It's time you checked in to see what on earth is going wrong. The best way to do this is via a comprehensive health assessment, which takes a really good look at why your hormones and vitamins aren't performing their functions and why your cells are grinding to a halt.

When Doreen, a 48 year-old highly anxious overworked lawyer with two grown up children, first came to see me she wasn't in good shape. She was exhausted and depressed, hadn't had a good night's rest for at least six months due to incessant hot flushes and yet somehow miraculously she managed to muddle her way through extremely demanding days at work without letting on that she was about to throw in the towel. Food was her comfort and her refuge. Despite her best instincts she couldn't help but give in to her sugar cravings and her desires for all those pastries and muffins that she knew just weren't good for her. After all, she had heard about the low carbohydrate diet but wondered how she'd be able to get through her day without her fix.

With her moods and her body in such disarray she didn't think it meant much that her hands and feet had become increasingly cold over the past year and she was even wearing bed socks in summer. Every night she would come home and studiously prepare the evening meal for her husband Dave without letting on that she was about to cave in. In fairness to Dave he was a little miffed that Doreen's desire for sex had evaporated but he merely put this down to the change of life. After all they had been married for twenty years.

One day when she finally had a 15-minute break in her schedule she decided it was time that she took matters into her own hands and what better way to do this than to go and see a doctor. Making sure that nobody noticed she sneaked out of the office and saw one doctor who prescribed sleeping pills, another suggested Prozac, which he said was really good for depression and menopausal problems, and finally another who offered her the latest treatment for HRT which he said might make her bloat a little but that was OK - she wouldn't notice as she was already overweight. She even tried the herbal remedy black cohosh but this didn't do much to relieve her distress.

How did she get through her day? Dragging herself out of bed at 6.30 a.m. as she had just got to sleep she gulped down a cup of coffee for breakfast, had another with a muffin when she got to work. Lunch was sandwiches on the run followed by a further cup of coffee. In the evenings she would often have a pasta dish or meat and vegetables meticulously prepared from a gourmet cook book capped off with a dessert like chocolate fudge ice cream or pecan pie, which would satisfy her desperate desire for that sweet fix. 2-3 glasses of wine, which helped her to unwind, would regularly accompany her evening meal and then amazingly she would have a final cup of coffee to round off her day.

Both of Doreen's parents had sustained heart attacks when they were quite young, her father at the age of 52 and her mother when she was 59. She didn't realise it but she was sitting on a time bomb just waiting to explode. If she didn't self-destruct, her genes would see to it that her flirtation with her own mortality would come to an untimely end. Through her own good fortune she'd heard that part of my practice was devoted to promoting wellness and dealing with women's problems.

As she could certainly do with a mountain of restoration and wasn't about to surrender to the scrap heap, she made an appointment to come and see me - on a Saturday naturally when she wasn't working. When she told me her story, which she did with lots of humour, which was quite astounding, I felt for her but was also quietly optimistic that there was much that could be achieved. I was greatly encouraged by Doreen's desire to not only regain her health and her passion for her husband, but also to avoid the same fate that tagged both of her parents. Even though she was nearly drained of all her vital energy she wasn't planning on developing any life-threatening illness in the future. She'd seen friends of her mother develop Alzheimer's dementia and become incapacitated due to osteoporosis and she was determined that this wouldn't happen to her. When Doreen asked me whether her predicament was familiar I nodded reassuringly. I was really looking forward to working with her as there was room for lots of improvement and I have seen so many women just like her who desperately wanted to feel better. I felt that there was a great deal that could be done with the right programme.

Before she presented to my surgery she was required to complete a comprehensive nutritional and health assessment. This is a very useful way to bring to light nutritional deficiencies and to find out which organs aren't performing at their best, based on a set of symptoms germane to these specific areas.

NUTRITIONAL ASSESSMENT

This revealed that she was lacking in the following nutrients:

- Vitamin A
- Vitamin B3
- Vitamin B6
- Vitamin C
- Essential fatty acids
- Magnesium
- Protein
- Acetylcholine

It's not unusual to have inadequate supplies of a number of nutrients so it didn't surprise me that the B vitamins, magnesium, essential fatty acids and protein were involved. Her diet, which was loaded with carbohydrates and lacking in essential protein, was abysmal. If you're regularly consuming muffins, candy bars, sandwiches, pastas and desserts and hardly any fish, lean meat, eggs, fruit or vegetables, not to mention the complete absence of any nuts, seeds or oils, you're going to be lacking in essential nutrients with protein, vitamins and fatty acids being at the top of that list. Excessive stress and her over-consumption of coffee, which is a diuretic, resulted in the depletion of some of the B vitamins and magnesium, which in turn made it more difficult for her to get a good night's sleep. Acetylcholine is a neurotransmitter, which is a brain chemical that facilitates memory, and she simply was not getting enough basic nutrition in order to make this chemical. I wondered how she managed to remember anything let alone cope with the demands of high-powered court cases and then get it together to look after her husband. If superwoman is fashioned on a shoestring she had to be close to the real deal.

ORGAN ASSESSMENT

The results of her questionnaire revealed that the following organs were not functioning optimally:

- The liver
- The adrenals
- Thyroid gland
- The ovaries

This was also not a major revelation. I had a sense that she was consuming more alcohol than was good for her liver. Her ovaries were winding down as she was negotiating the menopausal transition and her poor adrenals were failing to pick up the slack. With her demanding lifestyle she needed all the support she could get from her adrenals to at least provide her with some energy and they just weren't able to deliver. Cold extremities signalled that her thyroid was in trouble, which was another contributor to her ongoing fatigue.

To verify the above I ordered a complete hormonal panel together with a biochemical profile that targeted her risk factors for heart disease. To treat her hormonal imbalance, which was a key contributor to the state she was in, we needed to know what she was capable of producing. These were her results:

HORMONE PROFILE	REFERENCE RANGE
Oestradiol <80pmol/Litre	Postmenopausal< 160 pmol/Litre
Progesterone 1.3 nmol/Litre	Postmenopausal 0.0-2.7 nmol/Litre
DHEAS 1.3 Micromol/Litre	<11.7 micromol/Litre
Cortisol Morning Level 150 nmol/Litre	138-650 nmol/Litre
Cortisol Afternoon level 100nmol/Litre	70-325 nmol/Litre
Testosterone 2.5nmol/Litre	1-4.5 nmol/Litre
Melatonin 17.9pg/ml	10-40 pg/ml

Her decidedly low oestradiol levels strongly suggested that she was going through menopause. Her DHEA and cortisol levels were on the low side of normal, which confirmed that her adrenal glands were not keeping pace with the demands of her body. In addition to her B vitamin deficiencies, low cortisol and DHEA would be a primary explanation for her utter exhaustion. Melatonin is a hormone that is primarily produced at night and due to her poor sleeping habits her relatively normal levels were somewhat unexpected.

THYROID FUNCTION PANEL	REFERENCE RANGE
Free T3 3.05 pmol/Litre	2.5-6.0 pmol/Litre
Free T4 10.0 pmol/Litre	10-25 pmol/Litre
TSH 2.24 mIU/Litre	0.30-4.0 mIU/Litre

Although these levels are normal, they are on the low

side, indicating that Doreen was not producing enough thyroid hormones which would also contribute to her fatigue as well as her cold extremities.

GROWTH HORMONE ASSAY	REFERENCE RANGE
IGF 1 29 nmol/Litre	12-47 nmol/Litre

Measuring IGF 1 is the best way we have to assess growth hormone via a blood test. Doreen's IGF 1 level was quite reasonable and therefore it is more than likely that her growth hormone level was also satisfactory.

BIOCHEMICAL PROFILE	REFERENCE RANGE
Total cholesterol 5.6 nmol/Litre	3.0-5.5 nmol/Litre
Triglycerides 1.0 nmol/Litre	0.5-1.7 nmol/Litre
HDL 1.5 nmol/Litre	0.9-2.1 nmol/Litre
LDL 3.6 nmol/Litre	1.7-3.5 nmol/Litre
HS-CRP 3.0 mg/Litre	0.0-5.0 mg/Litre
Homocysteine 12 umol/Litre	5-12 umol/Litre
Lipoprotein (a) 0.69g/Litre	<0.30 g/Litre

This combination of results rang alarm bells as elevated total cholesterol, LDL and lipoprotein (a) together with HS-CRP and homocysteine being in the upper range of normal are all risk factors for heart disease. Aligned with a strong family history this needed urgent attention. We decided that it would be a good idea to organise further investigations of her cardiovascular system to establish whether she was in any immediate danger. I ordered a coronary CT scan, which is a simple test for the early detection of blocked arteries. What this scan does is identify calcium deposits in the blood vessels that supply the muscles of the heart. A high calcium score would suggest a reasonable amount of blockage, which might ultimately trigger a heart attack. Fortunately her calcium scores were extremely low.   As we wanted to leave nothing to chance she underwent a further cardiovascular test, which measured the degree of stiffness of her arteries and the efficiency of her heart muscle function.   This investigation was also normal which was very reassuring.   She appeared to be in no immediate risk of a catastrophe.

Her blood tests, which investigated gluten intolerance and candida infestation, were normal which was pleasing. The bone mineral density assessment was also within reasonable limits indicating no real danger of impending osteoporosis.   However, her hair mineral analysis which investigates the presence of toxic metals like lead, aluminium and mercury did show that she had elevated levels of mercury, and low levels of selenium and iodine which she needed to make her thyroid gland function effectively.

Once we knew that her hormones were low and she was lacking in vital nutrients all we had to do was to see how her cells were coming to terms with these deficiencies.   By performing those tests, which throw some light on the specifics of her cellular function, this allows us to plan her programme with more precision.   You can have all the hormones and vitamins in the world but if your cells aren't operating in the right environment then you'll feel unwell and lethargic and you won't know why.   These tests will tell you why. Standard blood tests won't. With inadequate supplies of hormones and vitamins, poor cellular activity would make it even more difficult for Doreen to get by.

BIO-IMPEDANCE ANALYSIS TEST

This investigation involves the attachment of electrodes to your feet and your hands to assess the electrical current flowing through your body, which is a very useful way to evaluate how efficiently your cells are functioning. Your cells need a certain amount of water to function, and this test can provide you with important information about your cellular hydration. Your body composition, including the distribution of your body fat and muscle tissue, can also be measured utilising this technology. As you age you tend to gain fat and lose muscle, which can lead to diabetes and heart disease.

Doreen's test revealed that she had an elevated fat mass and poor muscle mass, which reflected her lack of exercise. Her cellular hydration status was also below normal. All of these factors contributed to a low impedance index, which indicated that the electrical current wasn't flowing very efficiently through her body and that her cellular function was less than optimal. The low impedance index also indicated that her mitochondria or her cellular batteries weren't generating enough energy. Mitochondria are powered by antioxidants such as coenzyme Q10, vitamin E and alpha-lipoic acid.

BIOLOGICAL TERRAIN ASSESSMENT

This test assesses the acid/alkali balance of your cells, free radical levels and provides some clues as to how well your liver and adrenals are working. Your cells function within an optimum acid/alkali range. Too much acidity makes it more difficult for your cells to go about their daily business, which is to provide you with energy. Foods such as grains, alcohol, coffee and red meat are thought to increase acidity while all the fruits and vegetables especially the green vegetables create an alkaline environment. Doreen could easily be labelled the acid queen. Hardly a morsel of fruit or vegetables could be found on her plate while muffins, sandwiches and pasta occupied the lion's share of her daily sustenance. This resulted in her cells being far too acidic. Her free radical levels were elevated affirming that she needed antioxidant support and her adrenals were depleted. This supported the blood tests, which showed that her cortisol and DHEA levels were low.

'LIVE BLOOD CELL' ANALYSIS

By investigating the size, shape and association of your red cells, white cells and platelets as well as any abnormal cells that might be running around your blood stream this test can provide much more information. It can highlight nutrient deficiencies, detail the effects of unyielding free radical stress on your cells and show you how effectively your liver and digestive processes are operating. This is the kind of information that routine blood tests do not provide. Doreen's analysis revealed that she was deficient in vitamin B12, folic acid and essential fatty acids. Her liver also appeared to be dysfunctional and her cholesterol was under oxidative stress. Remember oxidised LDL is connected with the development of blocked arteries, which for Doreen spells trouble.

URINE ORGANIC ACID PROFILE

Your body is constantly undergoing metabolic reactions in order to generate energy. As a by-product of these reactions organic acids are formed. The excessive accumulation of these acids indicates that these processes are not running smoothly. They can be measured by collecting a urine sample allowing for the identification of specific nutrient deficiencies, depending upon which acids are elevated. Organic acids are also produced by intestinal bacteria and yeasts, which makes it possible to pinpoint imbalances of bowel germs and the kinds of infections that can promote ongoing health problems. This kind of investigation is very useful for establishing the underlying cause of fatigue, insomnia, clouded thinking and any other medical disorder that is not really managed in a satisfactory manner using conventional testing procedures.

Doreen's test confirmed that she had a deficiency of vitamins B2 and B3 as well as alpha-lipoic acid. Alpha-lipoic acid, a critical antioxidant, is used to help form a substance called acetyl-CoA which is then channelled into your body's primary energy producing cycle called the Krebb's cycle. She also had the build-up of an organic acid called succinate. Elevated succinate is a marker for deficiency of coenzyme Q10, the critical energy booster. The level of another organic acid called methylmalonyl-CoA was raised. This indicated vitamin B12 deficiency. Vitamin B12 is a very important nutrient for the functioning of your nervous system and sometimes your blood test might indicate that your levels of this vitamin are satisfactory and yet you may be suffering from a poor memory, moodiness and loss of balance for no apparent reason. This suggests that you might in fact have a deficiency of vitamin B12, which a standard blood test has failed to establish.

Finally she had elevated levels of 8-hydroxy-2'-deoxyguanosine (which is quite a mouthful) and also a product of oxidative damage to DNA, indicating that she was unquestionably suffering from the effects of excessive free radical stress. The beauty of this test is that it pinpoints very precisely which nutrients are needed to restore your cells to their energy producing best.

To summarise, there was ample evidence for Doreen's complete lack of vitality. Not only did she have low levels of oestradiol, DHEA, cortisol, thyroid hormones as well as very specific nutrient deficiencies, but her cells, which were having to operate in an unsympathetic acidic environment, were also wilting under the barrage of an unmerciless free radical onslaught, not to mention a liver and digestive system that were functioning way below their best. She also possessed a number of risk factors for heart disease including a contributory family history and elevated levels of lipoprotein (a), cholesterol and LDL as well as homocysteine and HS-CRP, which were in the danger zone. She was overweight to boot and ate far too many carbohydrates and not enough protein. You could argue that she was one stressed out lady who merely needed to improve her diet, have a holiday and get some treatment for her menopause but here we have very clearly defined metabolic and hormonal inadequacies that should respond very favourably to treatment which would make Doreen feel a whole lot better.

DOREEN'S PROGRAMME

Her diet certainly needed changing for openers. I suggested that she start her day a little earlier with a wholesome breakfast rather than gulping down a cup of coffee and racing off to work. Her breakfast plan included ½ cup of wholegrain cereal such as cornflakes purchased from a heath-food store, combined with LSA mix (linseed, sunflower seeds and almonds in the form of a fine powder) garnished with some walnuts, cashews and blueberries together with soymilk. I allowed her the pleasure of having one cup of coffee at work during her 11o'clock break but encouraged her to exchange this for a piece of fruit over time. I thought that the sandwiches she was having at lunchtime might be increasing her fatigue in the afternoon so I encouraged her to consume either fish such as tuna, sardines or salmon or white meat such as chicken or turkey with a salad. She could follow this with another cup of coffee if her need was overwhelming. In the evening I advised her to have foods that included protein such as fish, beans, white or lean meat with green vegetables and a salad and to reduce her consumption of pasta to twice weekly if she so desired. It goes without saying that the after dinner coffee was given the thumbs down.

Although she wasn't on a vitamin programme, her many deficiencies clearly indicated that she needed one.   I started her on a B vitamin complex with added selenium together with Memozeal the proprietary compound that I have formulated, which includes vitamin B12, folic acid, alpha-lipoic acid and an assortment of herbs to boost adrenal function. The B vitamins and folic acid would also hopefully lower her homocysteine levels.

To give her liver a lift, I suggested she commence a herbal tonic made up of st mary's thistle, dandelion and globe artichoke. With her essential fatty acid and magnesium deficiencies I thought it would be a good idea to initiate a formulation called Udo's choice (a compound devised by Canadian expert Udo Erasmus) which contains a mixture of omega 3, 6 and 9 fatty acids as well as magnesium diglycinate powder 400mg daily.   To deal with her need for coenzyme Q10, she started a supplement of this nutrient.

To reduce her elevated cholesterol and LDL levels I introduced policosanol and to combat raised lipoprotein (a) she had to take vitamin C, the amino acid L-lysine in the form of a powder and inositol hexanicotinate, the slow release form of niacin or vitamin B3. This protocol for managing lipoprotein (a) is described in chapter six. To minimise HS-CRP, which reflects inflammation, I advised her to consume ginger tea regularly and to include the herb curcumin in her cooking, as these are both anti-inflammatory herbs.

Finally, to address her hormonal problems, she commenced a combination of hormones in the form of a cream and was told to apply ½ gram of this formulation twice daily to her forearms.

This included:
- Triest 1mg/gram
- Progesterone 20mg/gram
- DHEA 15mg/gram

With regard to her low thyroid function, and to give her energy a further boost, a compounded thyroid formulation including 22.4 mcg of T4 and 6.8mcg of T3 was introduced.

I also suggested that she consider having her mercury fillings removed at some stage.

This might sound like a medicine chest full of remedies, which would make even the most accommodating of us rattle, but I was of the opinion that she needed an overhaul and she was optimistic about the new Doreen that might emerge from the embers of her metabolic and hormonal burn-out.

After three months she returned for a review. She had stuck to her diet, more or less, and was managing without her daily carbohydrate fix although she was still having 2-3 cups of coffee per day. The improvement in her energy was obvious and much to her relief she was finally getting some quality sleep. She had lost some weight, which considerably increased her enthusiasm for her programme. Her HS-CRP was markedly lower, her homocysteine had decreased to almost acceptable levels and her total cholesterol had also diminished. Her hormone levels had gone up but her DHEA, oestradiol and progesterone levels were still on the low side of normal so we decided just to bump up her progesterone to 40mg and her triest to 2mg daily. Her nutrient status indicated that she was no longer deficient in B vitamins or magnesium. Her free radical score on the BTA test was significantly lower, her liver was far less dysfunctional and her cells were less acidic. Her thyroid function test indicated that her hormone levels were now in mid-range.

On the down side, her LDL was still elevated as was her lipoprotein (a). I have found and I know other physicians have a similar experience, that it can be rather difficult to reduce lipoprotein (a). The supplement programme, which includes vitamin C, lysine and inositol hexanicotinate if adhered to over time, has the effect of neutralising any harmful effects of raised lipoprotein (a). Her needs for extra protein and essential fatty acids were still present as her nutritional assessment still indicated deficiencies of these.

I have often found that compromised digestive function can make it that much harder to assimilate essential nutrients. I suggested that she start off her day with a lemon squeezed into a cup of hot water. This stimulates digestive juices making it easier for Doreen to get full value from her nutritional programme.

With renewed vitality and rejuvenated cognitive powers Doreen had changed from a devastated demolition job to a turbocharged express, which breathed new life into her work situation and her relationship, for which her husband was eternally grateful.

As she was absolutely thrilled with the outcome so far, especially with the way she was feeling, we maintained the programme and scheduled a review for a further three months down the track.

It is now three years since Doreen commenced her programme and she is travelling admirably. She has remained on most of her supplements except for policosanol, as her cholesterol and LDL levels have diminished to totally acceptable levels. We've had to adjust her hormonal treatments from time to time. She has these reviewed on a three-monthly basis and, as her hot flushes returned with a vengeance before her most recent visit which was towards the end of 2003, we decided to change from creams to troches. She was fed-up with applying the cream to her arms every day and, by administering the troche under her tongue, it was possible to achieve more potent hormonal effects. So far so good as at the time of writing this section her hormones appear to be back on track.

Doreen's programme is a prototype of the kind of protocol that I have begun with a number of my patients for the past four years. Whilst there have been some spectacular successes with this initiative, like there was for Doreen, for others the changes have been more subtle. It does depend on your commitment to wellness and I have also found that the worse you are before you start this programme in terms of digestive complaints, fatigue, moodiness, poor memory, diminished sex drive and difficulties with losing weight the more perceptible will be your improvements.

An investigation that I believe will soon be the cornerstone of any wellness programme is an assay, which measures the micronucleus index. Your DNA undergoes constant repair and regeneration and a low micronucleus index indicates that this process is proceeding in a healthy fashion which means that your cells can continue to replicate effectively, whereas a high score indicates misrepair and excessive DNA damage, which is associated with ageing, and even increases the risk for such diseases as cancer and Alzheimer's disease.

Deficiencies of folate and magnesium increase the micronucleus index, as will drinking more than five cups of coffee or tea per day, which means that if these beverages are your poison you would need to indulge less. If your cells have to deal with excessive amounts of free radicals then your micronucleus index will also increase but the reassuring news is that supplementing with vitamins A, C, E, B12, folic acid and beta-carotene can decrease your score. (1)

I decided to test this out on some of my patients who are on the wellness programme and much to my delight all recorded a very low micronucleus index. These assays were performed by an organization called the CSIRO in Adelaide but it won't be long before this investigation becomes commercially available.

**These are the tests that I believe everyone who is
positively committed to their health should undergo:**

Your eternal health anti-ageing programme
• An analysis of your vitamin, mineral and protein deficiencies
• A comprehensive health appraisal of your organ function
• Measurement of all your hormones including growth hormone
• Bio-impedance analysis
• Biological terrain assessment
• 'Live blood cell' analysis
• Urinary organic acid profile
• Ultrafast CT scan of the heart
• Cardiovascular testing including evaluation of arterial stiffness and heart muscle function
• Hair mineral analysis
• Bone density assessment
• HDL/LDL Cholesterol
• Iron studies
• Liver function panel
• Prostate specific antigen
• HS-CRP
• Homocysteine and Lipoprotein (a)
• Thyroid hormone function including T3 and T4
• Candida and anti-gliadin antibodies
• Glucose/insulin metabolism

These investigations are all described in this book. If any of them are unfamiliar to you, then you can brush-up on your knowledge by reviewing the relevant section. Many people ask me when they should start this programme and I simply reply that there is no time like the present. The age range of those who have initiated the wellness programme in my clinic spans the late 20's to the late 70's. It is never too early but also never too late.

> **Everyone needs their hormones fine-tuned and I believe that everyone should be on a supplement programme. While this needs to be individualised, here is a list of all the supplements that I take which will provide you with a ball park idea of what you are looking at. For the record I've just turned 51.**

- Vitamin B complex 2 daily
- Vitamin E 200i.u.including mixed tocopherols and 50i.u. tocotrienols daily
- Vitamin C 1000mg daily
- Zinc 30mg daily
- Selenium 200mcg daily
- Magnesium diglycinate 400mg daily
- Memozeal 2 daily-this includes alpha-lipoic acid 200mg
- Acetyl-L-carnitine 2000mg daily
- Kelp 1000mg daily
- St mary's thistle 200mg daily
- Resveratrol 5mg daily
- Saw Palmetto 100mg daily
- Whey concentrate powder 20grms daily

- Rice protein concentrate 25grms daily
- Green powder 2 teaspoons daily-
  this contains wheat grass, barley greens and alfalfa
- Arthropro system one daily-this is a Life Extension Foundation formulation to limit inflammation
- Creatine powder 10grms daily
- Glucosamine sulphate 1000mg daily
- Chondroitin sulphate 400mg daily
- Quercetin 500mg daily
- Carnosine 500mg daily
- Glycerylphosphorylcholine 600mg daily
- DHEA 25mg daily
- Testosterone cream 30mg at night
- Progesterone cream 10mg at night
- Melatonin 3mg at night
- Trans-D tropin 15 drops daily Monday through till Friday
- Arimidex ½ tablet twice weekly

This is the regimen that has kept me going in good health and with lots of energy up to now. I'm a vegetarian so I have to augment with lots of protein. I don't take all the hormone treatments including DHEA, testosterone, progesterone, melatonin and trans-D tropin all the time, as I like to give my hormone receptors a break, which also allows for the manufacture of my own hormones. This is what I recommend to my patients. I also monitor my hormone levels every 3-6 months as I do with my patients, which also dictates whether I reduce supplementing with these. The progesterone helps to improve my sleep patterns and along with arimidex limits the amount of oestrogen that my body makes when I take DHEA.

Memozeal contains the herbs brahmi and gingko biloba and together with glycerylphosphorylcholine these are designed to boost my memory, which needs all the assistance it can get.

I take creatine to preserve my muscle mass and chondroitin and glucosamine sulphate because I jog and do regular weight training and these work to repair and maintain joints and cartilage. Arthropro systems is an anti-inflammatory agent and, aside from measuring HS-CRP, I believe it is a good idea to take this type of compound as a preventive in order to limit the potentially harmful effects of excess inflammation.

Carnosine is the antioxidant which binds heavy metal toxins and also prevents sugar that accumulates in the blood stream from coating protein, thereby possibly slowing down the ageing process. One of the primary events thought to govern ageing is the shortening of telomeres located at the end of your chromosomes. The chromosomes are your genetic material and the ability of your cells to replicate determines your ageing process. Once your telomeres start shortening ageing is postulated to set in. Carnosine has been shown to limit the shortening rate of telomeres, which might have life-extending potential. If you want more information on carnosine there is an article in the January 2001 edition of 'Life Extension,' which you can access via www.lef.org. Another excellent resource, which will provide you with objective scientific evidence about the benefits of carnosine and any other nutrient or hormone is Medline, accessible via the google search engine.

With exception to the hormones described in this programme you can use this protocol as an approximate template for the kind of regimen that might be appropriate for you but I do think that you should enlist the guidance of a health professional when you commence such an initiative.

I've said before that health and wellness are a gift and in these fragile times it behoves us more than ever to manage this gift with the utmost respect and care. I would encourage you not to take your health for granted and to commit to your wellness programme.

It will be a little while before technologies such as gene therapy, nanotechnology which involves the incorporation of small robots or nanobots to repair whatever damage is taking place in your body, stem cell and telemore therapy become available. Medicine's immediate future is accessible to all of us - utilising the best of medical technology and the benefits of natural remedies to allow you to become the healthiest person you can be.

BIBLIOGRAPHY

CHAPTER 2:

1. **Kopernik, G. and Shoham, Z.,** Tools for making correct decisions regarding hormone therapy.   Parts 1and 11, *Fertility and Sterility,* 2004; Jun; 81(6): 1458-1477.
2. **Dangour, A.D., Sibson, V.L, and Fletcher,** A. E., Hormones and supplements: Do they work? Micronutrient supplementation in later life: Limited evidence for benefit, *The Journal of Gerontology series A: Biological sciences and medical sciences,* 2004; 59: B659-B673.

CHAPTER 3:

1. **Barbieri, M., Rizzo, M.R. et al.,** Glucose regulation and oxidative stress in healthy centenarians, *Experimental Gerontology,* 2003; 38(1-2):137-43.
2. **Gruenewald, D.A. and Alvin M. Matsumoto,** A.M., Testosterone Supplementation Therapy for Older Men: Potential Benefits and Risks, *Journal of the American Geriatrics Society,* 2003; 51: (1): 101-115.
3. **Buneviciu, R., Kazanavicius, G., et al.,** Effects of thyroxine as compared with thyroxine plus triiodothyronine in patients with hypothyroidism, New England Journal of Medicine, 1999; 340(6): 424-429
4. **Brody, J.E., and Grady, D.,** *The New York Times guide to alternative health:* A consumer reference, Time Books: Henry Holt And Company, New York: 2001.
5. **Fletcher, R.H. and Fairfield, K.M.,** Vitamins for chronic disease in adults: clinical applications, *Journal of the American Medical Association,* 2002; 287 (23): 3127-3129.

CHAPTER 4:

1. **Thompson, J.L., Butterfield, G.E., et al.,** Effects of human growth hormone, insulin-like growth factor I, and diet and exercise on body composition of obese postmenopausal women, *Journal of Clinical Endocrinology and Metabolism,* 1998; 83(5): 147-184.
2. **Li, C., Samsioe, G., et al.,** Low-dose hormone therapy and carbohydrate metabolism, *Fertility and Sterility,* 2003; 79(3): 550-5.
3. **Kalish, G.M., Barrett-Connor, E., et al,** Association of endogenous sex hormones and insulin resistance among postmenopausal women: results from the Postmenopausal Estrogen/Progestin Intervention Trial, *Journal of Clinical Endocrinology and Metabolism,* 2003; 88(4): 1646-52.

CHAPTER 5:

1. **Richters, J., Grulich, A.E., et al,** Sex in Australia: sexual difficulties in a representative sample of adults, *Australia New Zealand Journal of Public Health,* 2003; 27 (2): 164-170.

2. **Becker, A.J., Ucker, S., et al,** Serum levels of human growth hormone during different penile conditions in the cavernous and systemic blood of healthy men and patients with erectile dysfunction, *Urology,* 2002; 59 (4): 609-614.

3. **Tsujimura, A., Matsumiya, K., et al,** Bioavailable testosterone with age and erectile dysfunction, *The Journal of Urology,* 2003; 170: 2345-2347.

4. **T'Sjoen, G., Goemaere, S., et al,** Perception of males' aging symptoms, health and well-being in elderly community-dwelling men is not related to circulating androgen levels, *Pyschoneuroendocrinology,* 2004; 29(2):   210-214.

5. **Modelska, K. and Cummings, S.,** Female sexual dysfunction in postmenopausal women: Systematic review of placebo-controlled trials, *American Journal of Obstetrics and Gynaecology,* 2003; 188: 286-293.

6. **Castelo-Branco, C., Blumel, J.E., et al,** Prevalence of sexual dysfunction in a cohort of middle-aged women: influences of menopause and hormone replacement therapy, *Journal of Obstetrics and Gynaecology,* 2003; 23(4): 426-430.

7. **Graziottin, A.,** Libido: the biologic scenario, 2000; 34 Suppl 1: S916.

8. **Lee, J.,** What you doctor may not tell you about menopause: The breakthrough book of natural progesterone, New York: Warner, 1996.

9. **Wren, B.G., Champion, S.M., et al.,** Transdermal progesterone and its effects on vasomotor symptoms, blood lipids, bone metabolic markers, moods and quality of life for postmenopausal women, *Menopause,* 2003; 10 (1): 138.

10. **Reiter, W.J., Pycha, A., et al.,** DHEA in the treatment of erectile dysfunction: a prospective double-blind randomized placebo-controlled study, *Urology,* 1999; 53(5): 590-594.

11. **Reiter, W.J., Pycha, A., et al.,** Serum DHEA sulphate concentration in men with erectile dysfunction, *Urology,* 2000; 55 (5): 755-758.

12. **Buvat, J.,** Androgen therapy with DHEA, *World Journal of Urology,* 2003; 21 (5): 346-355.

13. **Reiter, W.J. and Schatzl, G.,** DHEA in the treatment of erectile dysfunction in patients with different organic etiologies, *Urological Research,* 2001; 29(4): 278-281.

14. **Montorsi, F., Salonia A., et al,** The Ageing Male and erectile dysfunction, *World Journal of Urology,* 2002; 20: 283-285.

15. **Wespes, E.,** The Ageing penis, *World Journal of Urology* 2002; May 20 (1): 363-369.

16. **Stanislov, R., and Nikolova, V.,** Treatment of erectile dysfunction with pycnogenol and L-arginine, *Journal of Sexual and Marital Therapy*, 2003; 29(3): 207-213.

17. **Hong, B., Ji, Y.H., et al,** A double-blind crossover study evaluating the efficacy of Korean red ginseng in patients with erectile dysfunction: a preliminary report, *Journal of Urology,* 2002; 168(5): 207-213.

18. **Antoniou, L.D. and Shalhoub, R.,** Reversal of uraemic impotence by zinc, *Lancet,* 1977; 2(8044): 895-898.

19. **Xin, Z.C., Kim, E.K., et al,** Effects of icariin on cGMP-specific PDE5 and cAMP-specific PDE4 activities, *Asian Journal of Andrology,* 2003; 5(1): 151-158.

20. **Cherdshewasart, W. and Nimsakul, N.,** Clinical trials of Butea superba, an alternative herbal treatment for erectile dysfunction, *Asian Journal of Andrology,* 2003; 5(3): 243-246.

21. **Gonzales, G.F., Cordova, A., et al,** Effect of Lepimidium meyenii (MACA) on sexual desire and its absent relationship with serum testosterone in adult healthy men, *Andrologia,* 2002; 34(6): 367-372.

22. **Waynberg, J. and Brewer, S.,** Effects of Herbal vX on libido and sexual activity in premenopausal and postmenopausal women, *Advances and Therapeutics,* 2000; 17(5): 255-262.

23. **Brody, S.** High-dose ascorbic acid increases intercourse frequency and improves mood: a randomised controlled clinical trial, *Biological Psychiatry,* 2002; 15; 52(4): 371-374.

24. **Biagiotti, G. and Cavallini, G.,** Acetyl-L-carnitine vs. tamoxifen in the oral therapy of Peyronie's disease: a preliminary report, *British Journal of Urology International,* 2001; 88(1): 636-637.

25. **Prieto Castro, R.M., Leva Vallejo, M.E., et al,** Combined treatment with vitamin E and colchicines in the early stages of Peyronie's disease, *British Journal of Urology International,* 2003; 91(6): 522-524.

CHAPTER 6

1. **Santen, R.J.** Risk of breast cancer with progestins: critical assessment of current data, *Steroids,* 2003; 68: 953-964.

2. **Eden, J.,** Progestins and Breast cancer, *American Journal of Obstetrics and Gynaecology,* 2003; 188 (5): 1123-1131.

3. **Kuhl, H.** Mechanisms of sex steroids; future developments, *Maturitas,* 2004; 15; 47(4): 285-291.

4. **Sitruk-Ware, R.,** Pharmacologic profile of progestins, *Maturitas,* 2004; 47: 277-282.
5. **De lignieres, B.,** Effects of progestogens on the postmenopausal breast, *Climacteric,* 2002; 5: 229-235.
6. **De lignieres, B., De Vathaire, F., et al,** Combined hormone replacement therapy and risk of breast cancer in a French cohort study of 3175 women, *Climacteric,* 2002; 5: 332-340.
7. **Formby, B., and Wiley, T. S.** Progesterone inhibits growth and induces apoptosis in breast cancer cells; Inverse effects on Bcl-2 and p53, *Annals of Clinical and Laboratory Science,* 1998; 28 (6): 360-366.
8. **Archer, D, F., Dorin M., et al,** Effects of lower doses of conjugated equine estrogens and medroxyprogesterone acetate on endometrial bleeding, *Fertility and Sterility,* 2001; 75(6): 1080-1087.
9. **Utian, W. H., Shoupe, D., et al,** Relief of vasomotor symptoms and vaginal atrophy with lower doses of conjugated equine estrogens and medroxyprogesterone acetate. *Fertility and Sterility,* 2001; 75 (6): 1065-1079.
10. **Watts, N. B., Notelovitz, M., et al,** Comparison of oral estrogens and estrogens plus androgen on bone mineral density, menopausal symptoms, and lipid-lipoprotein profiles in surgical menopause, *Obstetrics and Gynecology,* 1995; 85: 529-537.
11. **Husband, A.R.,** Red Clover isoflavone supplements: safety and pharmacokinetics, *Journal of the British Menopause Society,* Supplement S1, 2001: 4-7.
12. **Kronenburg F. and Fugh-Berman, A.,** Complementary and alternative medicine for menopausal symptoms: a review of randomised control trials, *Annals of Internal Medicine,* 2002; 19, 137 (10): 805-813.
13. **Chen, Y.M., Ho, S.C., et al,** Soy isoflavones have a favourable effect on bone loss in Chinese postmenopausal women with lower bone mass; a double-blind, randomized, controlled trial, *Journal of Clinical Endocrinology and Metabolism,* 2003; 88(10): 4740-4747.
14. **Persky, V.W. and Turyk, M.E.,** Effect of soy protein on endogenous hormones in postmenopausal women, *American Journal of Clinical Nutrition,* 2002; 75(1): 145-153.
15. **Nestel, P.,** Isoflavones and cardiovascular function, *Journal of the British Menopause Society,* Supplement S1, 2001; 12-16.
16. **Woodside, J.,** Isoflavones and breast cancer, *Journal of the British Menopause Society,* Supplement S1, 2001; 17-21.
17. **Messina, M., Gardner, C., and Barnes,** S., Fourth International symposium on the role of soy in preventing and treating chronic disease, *Journal of Nutrition,* 2002; 132: 547S-551S.

18. **Chiechi, L.M., Secreto, G., et al,** Efficacy of a soy rich diet in preventing postmenopausal osteoporosis: the Menfis randomized trial, *Maturitas,* 2002; 30, 42(4): 295-230.

19. **Klevay, L.M. and Wildman, R.E.,** Meat diets and fragile bones. *Journal of Trace Elements and Medical Biology,* 2002; 16(3): 149-154.

20. **Lean, M.J., Julie T., Davies, J.T., et al,** A crucial role for thiol antioxidants in estrogen-deficiency bone loss, *Journal of Clinical Investigations,* 2003; 112: 915-923.

21. **Fiattarone Singh, M.F.,** Physical activity and bone health, *Australian Family Physician,* 2004; 33 (3): 125.

22. **Riggs, B.L, Khosla, S., and Melton, L.J.,** Sex steroids and the construction and conservation of the adult skeleton, *Endocrine Reviews,* 2002; 23 (3): 279-302.

23. **Pfeilschifter, J., Koditz, R., et al,** Changes in proinflammatory cytokine activity after menopause, *Endocrine reviews,* 2002; 23(1): 90-119.

24. **Watts, N.B., Notelovitz, M., et al,** Comparison of oral estrogens and estrogens plus androgens on bone mineral density, menopausal symptoms and lipoprotein profiles, *Menopause Obstetrics and Gynecology,* 1995; 85(4): 529-537.

25. **Takayanagi, R., Goto, K., et al,** DHEA as a possible source for estrogen formation in bone cells; correlation between bone mineral density and serum DHEA-sulfate concentration in postmenopausal women and the presence of aromatase to be enhanced by 1,25 dihydroxyvitamin D3 in human osteoblasts, *Mechanisms of Ageing and Development* 2002; 123(8): 1107-1114.

26. **Seeman, E., and Eisman, J.A.,** Treatment of osteoporosis: why, whom, when and how to treat, *Medical Journal of Australia,* 2004; 180(6): 298-303.

CHAPTER 7

1. **Clemons, M., and Paul Goss, P.,** Estrogen and the risk of breast cancer, *New England of Medicine,* 2001; 344(4): 276-285.

2. **Warren, M.P.,** A comparative review of the risks and benefits of hormone replacement therapy regimens, *American Journal of Obstetrics and Gynecology,* 2004; 190(4): 1141-1167.

3. **Yue, W., Stanten, R.J., et al,** Genotoxic metabolites of oestradiol in breast: potential mechanisms of estradiol induced carcinogenesis, *Journal of Steroid biochemistry and Molecular Biology,* 2003; 86: 477-486.

4. **Rogan, E.R., Badawi A.F., et al,** Relative imbalances in estrogen metabolism and conjugation in breast tissue of women with carcinoma: potential biomarkers of susceptibility to cancer, *Carcinogenesis,* 2003; 24(4): 697-702.

3. **Samuni, A.M., Chaung, E.Y., et al,** Semiquinone radical intermediate in catechol estrogen-mediated cytotoxicity and mutagenesis: Chemoprevention strategies with antioxidants, *Proceedings of the National Academy of Science,* 2003;100(9): 5390-5395.

6. **Hari, K., Bhat, H.K., Calaf, G., et al,** Critical role of oxidative stress in estrogen-induced carcinogenesis, *Proceedings of the National Academy of Science,* 2003; 100(7): 3913-3918.

7. **Jernstrom, H., Klug, T.L., et al,** Predictors of the plasma ratio of 2-hydroxyestrone to 16 alpha-hydroxyestrone among pre-menopausal, nulliparous women from four ethnic groups, *Carcinogenesis,* 2003; 24(5): 991-1005.

8. **Pasqualini, J.R., and Chetrite,** G., Paradoxical effect of estradiol: it can block its own biotransformation in human breast cancer cells, *Journal of Steroid Biochemistry and Mol. Biology,* 2001; 78(1): 21-24.

9. **Anderson, G.L., Limacher, M., et al,** Effects of conjugated equine oestrogen in postmenopausal women with hysterectomy: the Women's Health Initiative Randomised Control Trial, *Journal of the American Medical Association,* 2004; 291(14): 1701-1712.

10. **Song, R.X., and Santen, R.J.,** Apoptotic actions of estrogen, *Apoptosis,* 2003; 8(1): 55-60.

11. **Stoll, B.A.,** Dietary supplements of dehydroepiandrosterone in relation to breast cancer risk, *European Journal of Clinical Nutrition,* 1999; 53(10): 771-775.

12. **Rohr, U.D.,** The impact of testosterone imbalance on depression and women's health, *Maturitas,* 2002; 41 Suppl 1: S25-46.

13. **Renehan, A.G., Zwahlen, M., et al,** Insulin-like growth factor (IGF)-1 IGF binding protein-3, and cancer risk: systematic review and meta-regression analysis, *Lancet* 2004; 363: 1346-1353.

14. **Onland-Moret, N.C., Kaaks, R., et al,** Urinary endogenous sex hormone levels and the risk of postmenopausal breast cancer, *British Journal of Cancer,* 2003; 88 (9): 1394-1399.

15. **Cui, X., Lazard, Z., et al,** Progesterone crosstalks with insulin-like growth factor signalling in breast cancer cells via induction of insulin receptor substrate-2, *Oncogene,* 2003; 22(44): 6937-6941.

16. **Thomas, T., Rhodin, J., et al,** Progestins initiate adverse events of menopausal estrogen therapy, *Climacteric,* 2003; 6(4): 293-301.

17. **Zhu, B.T.,** Medical hypothesis: hyperhomocysteinemia is a risk factor for estrogen-induced hormonal cancer, *International Journal of Oncology,* 2003; 22(3): 499-508.

18. **Zhang, S.M., Willett, W.C., et al,** Plasma folate, vitamin B6, vitamin B12, homocysteine, and risk of breast cancer, *Journal of the National Cancer Institute,* 2003; 95(5): 373-380.

19. **Semenza, J.C., Delfino, R.J., et al,** Breast cancer risk and methylenetetrahydrofolate reductase polymorphism, *Breast Cancer Research and Treatment,* 2003; 77(3): 217-223.

20. **Dai, Q., Shu, X.O., et al,** Consumption of animal foods, cooking methods, and risk of breast cancer, *Cancer Epidemiology Biomarkers and Prevention,* 2002; (9): 801-808.

21. **Sinha, R.,** An epidemic approach to studying heterocyclic amines, *Mutation Research* 2002; Sep 30, 506-507.

22. **Cho, E., Spiegelman, D., et al,** Premenopausal fat intake and risk of breast cancer, *Journal of the National Cancer Institute* 2003; 95(14): 1079-1085.

23. **Food, nutrition and the prevention of cancer:** a global perspective. Banta Book group: Menasha 1997.

24. **Shin, M.H., Holmes, M.D., et al,** Intake of dairy products, calcium, and vitamin D and risk of breast cancer, *Journal of the National Cancer Institute,* 2002; 94(17): 1301-1311.

25. **Outwater, J.L., Nicholson, A., et al,** Dairy products and breast cancer: the IGF-1, estrogen and bGH hypothesis, *Medical Hypothesis,* 1997; 48(6): 453-461.

26. **Knekt, P., Jarvinen, R., et al,** Intake of dairy products and the risk of breast cancer, *British Journal of Cancer,* 1996; 73(5): 687-691.

27. **Holmes, M.D., Liu, S., et al,** Dietary carbohydrates, fiber, and breast cancer risk, *American Journal of Epidemiology,* 2004; 159(8): 732-739.

28. **Key, T.J., Appleby, P.N., et al,** Body mass index, serum sex hormones, and breast cancer risk in postmenopausal women, *Journal of the National Cancer Institute,* 2003; (16): 1218-1226.

29. **Stoll, B.A.,** Upper abdominal obesity, insulin resistance and breast cancer risk, *International Journal of Obesity and Related Metabolic Disorders,* 2002; 26(6): 747-753.

30. **Mitra, S., Faruque, F.S., and Avis, A.L.,** Breast cancer and environmental risk: where is the link, J*ournal of Environmental Health,* 2004; 66(7): 24-32.

31. **Gammon, M.D., Wolff, M.S., et al,** Environmental toxins and breast cancer on Long Island 11. Organochlorine compound levels in blood, *Cancer Epidemiology, Biomarkers and Prevention,* 2002; (8): 686-697.

32. **Martin, M.B., Reiter, R., et al,** Estrogen-like activity of metals in MCF-7 breast cancer cells, *Endocrinology,* 2003; 144(6): 242-255.

33. **Velicer, C.M., Heckbert, S.R., et al,** Antibiotic use in relation to the risk of breast cancer, *Journal of the American Medical Association,* 2004; 292(7): 827-835.

34. **Goss, P.E.,** Breast cancer prevention-clinical trials strategies involving aromatase inhibitors, *Journal of Steroid Biochemistry and Molecular Biology,* 2003; (86): 487-493.

35. **Shin-ichi, H., Sakamoto, T., et al,** Estrogen and growth factor signalling pathway: basic approaches for clinical application, *Journal of Steroid Biochemistry and Molecular Biology,* 2003; 86: 433-442.

36. **Rohr, U.D., and Herold, J.,** Melatonin deficiencies in women, *Maturitas,* 2002; 41 Suppl 1: S85-104.

37. **Gonzalez-Sancho, J.M., Figueroa, A., et al,** Inhibition of proliferation and expression of T1 and cyclin D1 genes by thyroid hormone in mammary epithelial cells, *Molecular Carcinogenesis,* 2002; 1: 25-34.

38. **Lee, J.R., Zava, D., and Hopkins, V.,** What your doctor may not tell you about breast cancer. How hormone balance can help save your life. New York: Penguin Putnam Inc, 2002.

39. **Malet, C., Spritzer, P., et al,** Progesterone effect on cell growth, ultrastructural aspect and estradiol receptors of normal human breast epithelial cell culture, *Journal of Steroid Biochemistry and Molecular Biology,* 2000; 73(3-4): 171-181.

40. **Foidart, J.M., Colin C., et al,** Estradiol and progesterone regulate the proliferation of human epithelial cells, *Fertility and Sterility* 1998; 69(5): 963-969.

41. **Cui, X., Lazard, Z., et al,** Progesterone crosstalks with insulin-like growth factor signalling in breast cancer cells via induction of insulin receptor substrate-2, *Oncogene,* 2003; 22(44): 6737-6741.

42. **Medina, R.A., Meneses, A.M., et al,** Estrogen and progesterone up-regulate glucose transporter expression in ZR-75-1 human breast cancer cells, *Endocrinology,* 2003; 144(10): 4527-4535.

43. **Olsson, H.L., Ingvar, C., Bladstrom, A.,** Hormone replacement therapy containing progestins and given continuously increases breast carcinoma risk in Sweden, *Cancer,* 2003; 97: 1387-1392.

44. **Zhang, S.M.,** Role of vitamins in the risk, prevention and treatment of breast cancer, *Current Opinions in Obstetrics and Gynecology,* 2004 Feb; 16 (1): 19-25.

45. **Holick, M.F.,** Vitamin D: importance in the prevention of cancers, type1 diabetes, heart disease and osteoporosis, *American Journal of Clinical Nutrition,* 2004, 79(3): 362-371.

46. **Stripp, C., Overad, K.,** et al, Fish intake is positively associated with breast cancer incidence rate, *The Journal of Nutrition,* 2003; 133(11): 3664-3669.

47. **Wu, A.H., Tseng, C.C.,** et al, Tea Intake, COMT Genotype, and Breast Cancer in Asian-American women, *Cancer Research,* 2003; 63: 7526-7529.

48. **Stoner, G., Casto, B.,** et al, Development of a multi-organ rat model for evaluating chemopreventive agents: efficacy of indole-3 carbinol, *Carcinogenesis,* 2002; 23(2): 265-272.

49. **Auborn, K.F., Fan, S.,** et al, Indole-3 carbinol is a negative regulator of oestrogen, *Journal of Nutrition, 2003;* 133 (7 Suppl): 2470S-2475S.

50. **Pisani, P., and Forman, D.,** Declining mortality from breast cancer in Yorkshire, 1983-1998, extent and causes, *British Journal of Cancer,* 2004; 90(3): 652-656.

51. **De Koning, H.J.,** Mammographic screening: evidence from randomised controlled trials, *Annals of Oncology,* 2003; 8: 1185-1189.

52. **Saputo, L.,** Beyond Mammography, *Townsend Letter for Doctors and Patients,* 2004; 251: 65-68.

53. **Collins, A., and Yuan, L.,** Overexpression of the MT1 melatonin receptor in MCF-7 human breast cancer cells inhibits mammary tumour formation in nude mice, *Cancer Letters,* 2003; 189 (1): 49-57.

54. **Sanchez-Barcelo, E.J., Cos S.,** et al, Melatonin and mammary cancer: a short review, *Endocrine Related Cancer,* 2003; (2): 153-159.

55. **Cos, S., Mediavilla, M.D.,** et al, Does melatonin induce apoptosis in MCF-7 human breast cancer cells in vitro? *Journal of Pineal Research,* 2002; 32(2): 90-96.

56. **Cos, S., Mediavilla, M.D.,** et al, Melatonin increases P53 and P21 WAF1 expression in MCF-7 human breast cancer cells in vitro, *European Journal of Life Sciences,* 1999; 65(4): 415-420.

57. **Lissoni, P., Barni, S.,** et al, Decreased toxicity and increased efficacy of cancer chemotherapy using the pineal hormone melatonin in metastatic solid tumours with poor clinical status, *European Journal of Cancer,* 1999; 35(12): 1688-1692.

58. **Bizzani, M., and Cucina, A.,** Melatonin and Vit D3 increase TGF-beta1 release and induce growth inhibition in breast cancer cell cultures. *Journal of Surgical Research* 2003; 110(2): 332-337.

59. **Rao, G.N., Ney, E., Herbert, R.A.,** Effect of melatonin and linoleic acid on mammary cancer in transgenic mice with C-neu breast cancer, *Oncogene, Breast Cancer Research and Treatment,* 2000; 64(3): 287-296.

60. **Labrie, F., Luu-The, V., et al,** Endocrine and intracrine sources of androgens in women: inhibition of breast cancer and other roles of androgens and their precursor dehydroepiandrosterone, *Endocrine Review,* 2003; 24(2): 152-82.

61. **Norman, H.A., and Butrum, R. R.,** The role of dietary supplements during cancer therapy, *The Journal Of Nutrition,* 2003; 133: 3794S-3799S.

62. **Conklin, K. A.,** Dietary antioxidants during cancer chemotherapy: Impact on chemotherapeutic effectiveness and development of side effects, *Nutrition and Cancer,* 2000; 37(1): 1-18.

63. **Prasad, K.N., Cole, W.C., et al,** Pros and cons of antioxidant use during radiation therapy, *Cancer Treatment Reviews,* 2002; 28: 79-91.

64. **Prasad, K.N., Cole, W.C., et al,** Scientific Rationale for using High-Dose multiple micronutrients as an adjunct to standard and experimental cancer therapies, *Journal of the American College of Nutrition,* 2001; 20(5): 450S-463S.

65. **Lesperance, M.L, Olivotto, I.A., et al,** Mega-dose vitamins and minerals in the treatment of non-metastatic breast cancer: an historical cohort study, *Breast Cancer Research and Treatment,* 2002; 76(2): 137-143.

66. **Fleischauer, A.T., Simonsen, N., and Arab., L.,** Antioxidant supplements and risk of breast cancer recurrence and breast cancer-related mortality among postmenopausal women, *Nutrition and Cancer,* 2003; 46(1): 15-22.

67. **Jiang, C., Ganther, H., and Lu J.,** Monomethyl selenium-specific inhibition of MMP-2 and VEGF expression: implications for angiogenic switch regulation, *Journal of Molecular Carcinogenesis,* 2000; 29(4): 236-50.

68. **Choi, J.A., Kim, J.Y.,** Induction of cell cycle arrest and apoptosis in human breast cancer cells by quercetin, *International Journal of Oncology,* 2001; 19(4): 837-844.

69. **Colston, K. W., Hansen, C.M.,** Mechanisms implicated in the growth regulatory effects of vitamin D in breast cancer, *Endocrine Related Cancer,* 2002; 9(1): 45-59.

70. **Welsh, J., Wietzke, J.A., et al,** Vitamin D-3 receptor as a target for breast cancer prevention, *Journal of Nutrition,* 2003; 133(7 Suppl): 2425S-2433S.

71. **Hussain, E.A., Mehta, R.R., et al,** Efficacy and mechanism of action of 1alpha-hydroxy-24-ethyl-cholecalciferol (1alpha[OH]D5) in breast cancer prevention and therapy, *Recent Results in Cancer Research,* 2003; 164: 393-411.

72. **Yu, W., Sanders, B.G. and Kline, K.,** RRR-alpha-tocopherol succinate-induced apoptosis of human breast cancer cells involves Bax translocation to mitochondria, *Cancer Research,* 2003; 63(10): 248-391.

73. **Czeczuga-Semeniuk, E., Wolczynski, S., et al,** Cell 13-cis retinoic acid and all-trans retinoic acid in the regulation of the proliferation and survival of human breast cancer cell line MCF-7, *Cellular and Molecular Biology Letters,* 2001; 6 (4): 925-939.

74. **Lycopene.** Monograph, *Alternative Medicine Review,* 2003; 8(3): 336-42.

75. **Calcium-D-glucarate.** Monograph. *Alternative Medicine Review,* 2002; 7(4): 336-339.

76. **Kodama, N., Komuta, K., and Nanba, H.,** Can maitake MD-fraction aid cancer patients, *Alternative Medicine Review,* 2002; 7(3): 236-239.

77. **Somasundaram, S., Edmund, N.A., et al,** Dietary curcumin inhibits chemotherapy-induced apoptosis in models of human breast cancer, *Cancer Research,* 2002; 62 (13): 3868-3875.

78. **Makridakis, N.M., and Reichardt, J.K.,** Molecular epidemiology of androgen-metabolic loci in prostate cancer: predisposition and progression, *Journal of Urology,* 2004; 171(2 Pt 2): S25-29.

79. **Schulz, W.A., Burchardt, M., and Cronauer, M.V.,** Molecular biology of prostate cancer, *Molecular Human Reproduction,* 2003; 8: 437-448.

80. **Bosland, M.C.,** The role of steroid hormones in prostate cancer, *Journal of the National Cancer Institute,* 2000; Monographs No 27: 39-66.

81. **Kaufman, J. M.,** The effect of androgen supplementation therapy on the prostate, *The Aging Male,* 2003; 6: 166-174.

82. **Stas, S. N., Anastasiadis, A. G., et al,** Urologic aspects of andropause, *Urology,* 2003; (61): 261-266.

83. **Testosterone and Aging:** Clinical research directions. Washington, D.C. The National Academies Press, 2004.

84. **Ntais, C., Polycarpou, A., and Tsatsoulis, A.,** Molecular epidemiology of prostate cancer: androgens and polymorphisms in androgen-related genes, *European Journal of Endocrinology,* 2003; (149): 469-477.

85. **Rhoden, E.L., and Morgentaler, A.,** Testosterone replacement in

hypogonadal men at high risk for prostate cancer: results of 1-year treatment in men with prostatic intraepithelial neoplasia, *Journal of Urology* 2003; Dec: 170 (6 Pt1): 2348-2351.

86. **Schatzl, G., Madersbacher, S., et al,** Associations of serum testosterone with microvessel density, androgen receptor density and androgen receptor gene polymorphism in prostate cancer, *Journal of Urology*, 2003; 169(4): 1312-1315.

87. **Renehan, A.G., Zwahlen, M., et al,** Insulin-like growth factor (IGF)-1, IGF binding protein-3, and cancer risk: systematic review and meta-regression analysis, *Lancet,* 2004; 363(9418): 1346-1353.

88. **Holly, J.M.P., Gunnell, D.J., and Davey Smith, G.,** Growth hormone, IGF-1 and cancer. Less intervention to avoid cancer? More intervention to prevent cancer? *Journal of Endocrinology,* 1999; 162: 321-330.

89. **Du Pan, M.,** Are the hormones of youth carcinogenic? *Annals of Endocrinology* (Paris), 1999; 60(5): 392-397.

90. **The DHEA debate:** A critical review of clinical and experimental data. *Life Extension Magazine* March 2004; 21-40.

91. **Rodriguez, C., McCullogh, M.L., et al,** Calcium, dairy products and risk of prostate cancer in a prospective cohort of United States men, *Cancer Epidemiology Biomarkers and Prevention,* 2003; 12: 597-603.

92. **Chan, J.M., Stampfer, M.J., et al,** Dairy products, calcium and prostate cancer risk in the Physicians health study, *American Journal of Clinical Nutrition,* 2001; 74(4): 549-554.

93. **Qin, L.Q., Wang, P.Y., et al,** Estrogen: one of the risk factors in milk for prostate cancer, *Medical Hypothesis,* 2004; 62(1): 133-142.

94. **Leitzmann, M., Stampfer, M.J., et al,** Zinc supplementation use and risk of prostate cancer, *Journal of the National Cancer Institute,* 2003; 95(13): 1004-1007.

95. **Heinonen, O., Albanes, D., et al,** Prostate cancer and supplementation with alpha tocopherol and ß-carotene: incidence and mortality in a controlled trial, *Journal of the National Cancer Institute,* 1998; 90: 440-446.

96. **Sharpe C. R. and Siematycki, J.,** Case-control study of alcohol consumption and prostate cancer risk in Montreal, Canada, *Journal of Cancer Causes and Control* 2001; 12: 589-598.

97. **Sesso, H.D., Paffenberger, R.S., Jr, and Lee, I.M.,** Alcohol consumption and risk of prostate cancer: The Harvard Alumni Health Study, *International Journal of Epidemiology,* 2001; 304: 749-755.

98. **Ritchie, J.M., Vial, S.L., et al,** Organochlorines and risk of prostate cancer, *Journal of Occupational and Environmental Medicine,* 2003; 45(7): 692-702.

99. **Pukkala, E., Aspholm, R., et al**, Incidence of cancer among Nordic airline pilots over five decades: occupational cohort study, *British Medical Journal*, 2002; 14, 325(7364): 567.

100.**Thompson, I.M, Pauler, D.K., et al,** Prevalence of Prostate cancer among men with a prostate-specific antigen level less than/equal 4.0ng/ml, *New England Journal of Medicine*, 2004; 350(22): 2239-2264.

101.**Schmidt, H, P., Reisen, W., and Prikler, L.**, Update on screening for prostate cancer with prostate-specific antigen, *Critical Reviews in Oncology/Haematology*, 2004; (50): 71-78.

102.**Ian, M., Goodman, P. J., et al,** The Influence of Finasteride on the Development of Prostate Cancer, *The New England Journal of Medicine*, 2003; 349(3): 215-224.

103.**Djavan, B., Zlotta, A., et al,** Chemotherapeutic preventive strategies for prostate cancer, *The Journal of Urology*, 2004; 171(2, part 2 of 2): S10-S13.

104.**Wilkinson, S., and Chodak, G. W.**, Critical review of complementary therapies for prostate cancer, *Journal of Clinical Oncology*, 2003; 21(11): 2199-2210.

105.**Hebert, J. R., Hurley, T.G., et al,** Nutritional and socio-economic factors in relation to prostate cancer mortality: a Cross-national study, *Journal of the National Cancer Institute*, 1998; 90: 1637-1647.

106.**Osaka, K, Nakao, M., et al,** Serum phytoestrogens and prostate cancer risk in a nested case-control study among Japanese men, *Cancer Science*, 2004; 95(1): 65-71.

107.**Li, H., Stampfer, M. J., et al,** A prospective study of plasma selenium levels and prostate cancer risk, *Journal of the National Cancer Institute*, 2004; 96: 696-703.

108.**Reported in Wilkinson, S., and Chodak, G. W.**, Critical review of complementary therapies for prostate cancer, *Journal of Clinical Oncology*, 2003; 21 (11): 2199-2210.

109.**Klein, E. A.**, Selenium: Epidemiology and basic science, *The Journal of Urology*, 2004; 171(2, Part 2): S50.

110.**Terry, P. D., Rohan, T. E., and Wolk, A.**, Intakes of fish and marine fatty acids and the risks of cancers of the breast and prostate and of other hormone-related cancers: a review of the epidemiologic evidence *American Journal of Clinical Nutrition*, 2003; 77(3): 532-543.

111. **Howells, L. M., Gallacher-Horley, B., Catherine, E.**, Indole-3 carbinol inhibits protein kinase B/Akt and induces apoptosis in the human breast tumor cell line MDA MB468 but not in the nontumorigenic HBL100 line, *Molecular Cancer Therapeutics*, 2002; 1: 1161-1172.

112. Le, H. T., Schaldach, C.M., et al, Plant-derived 3, 3'-diindolylmethane is a strong androgen antagonist in human prostate cancer cells, *Journal of Biological Chemistry,* 2003; 278(23): 21136-21145.

113. Ho, E., Boileau, T.W., and Bray, T.M., Dietary influences on endocrine-inflammatory interactions in prostate cancer development, *Archives of Biochemical Biophysics,* 2004; 428; (1): 109-117.

114. Gao, S., Liu, G. Z. S., and Wang, Z., Modulation of androgen receptor-dependent transcription by resveratrol and genistein in prostate cancer cells, *Prostate,* 2004; 59(2): 214-215.

115. Xi, S. C., Siu, S. W., et al, Inhibition of androgen-sensitive LNCaP prostate cancer growth in vivo by melatonin: association of antiproliferative action of the pineal hormone with mt1 receptor protein expression, *Prostate,* 2001; 46(1): 52-61.

116. Shiu, S.Y., Law, I.C., et al, Melatonin slowed the early biochemical progression of hormone refractory prostate cancer in a patient whose prostate tumour tissue expressed MT1 receptor subtype, *Journal of Pineal Research,* 2003; 35(3): 177-182.

117. Rimler, A., Culig, Z., et al, Nuclear exclusion of the androgen receptor by melatonin, *Journal of Steroid Biochemistry and Molecular Biology,* 2002; 81: 77-84.

118. Kristal A. R., Vitamin A, retinoids and carotenoids as chemopreventive agents for prostate cancer, *The Journal of Urology,* 2004; 171(2, part 2 of 2): S54-S58.

119. Schernhammer, E.S., Laden, F., et al, Night-shift work and risk of colorectal cancer in the nurses' health study, *Journal of the National Cancer Institute,* 2003; 95(11): 825-828.

120. Jedrychowski, W., Steindof, K., et al, Alcohol consumption and the risk of colorectal cancer at low levels of micronutrient intake, *Medical Science Monitor* 2002; 8(5): 357-363.

121. Soliman, A.S., Smith, M.A., et al, Serum organochlorine pesticide levels in patients with colorectal cancer in Egypt, *Archives of Environmental Health,* 1997; 52(6): 409-415.

122. Shaheen, N.J., Silverman, L.M., et al, Association between hemochromatosis gene mutation carrier status and the risk of colon cancer, *Journal of the National Cancer Institute,* 2003; 85: 154-159.

123. Poullis, A., Foster, R., et al, Bowel inflammation as measured by fecal calprotectin: a link between lifestyle factors and colorectal cancer risk, *Cancer Epidemiology Biomarkers and Prevention,* 2004; 13(2): 279-284.

124. Erlinger, T., Platz, E. A., et al, C-reactive protein and the risk of

incidental colorectal cancer, *Journal of the American Medical Association,* 2004; 291(5): 585-590.

125.**Slattery, M.L., Levin T.R., et al,** Family history and colorectal cancer: predictors of risk, *Cancer Causes and Control,* 2003; 14(9): 879-887.

126.**Hawk, E.T., Umar, A., and Viner, J.L.,** Colorectal cancer chemoprevention-an overview of the science, *Gastroenterology,* 2004; 126(5): 1423-1444.

127.**Kohno, H., Yasui, Y., et al,** Dietary seed oil-rich in conjugated linolenic acid from bitter melon inhibits azoxymethane-induced rat colon carcinogenesis through elevation of colonic PPARgamma expression and alteration of lipid composition, *International Journal of Cancer* 2004; 110(6): 896-901.

128.**Tsuda, H., Sekine, K., et al,** Prevention of colon carcinogenesis and carcinoma metastasis by orally administered bovine lactoferrin in animals, *Biofactors,* 2000; 12(14): 83-88.

129.**Belobrajdic, D., Mcintosh, G.H., Owens, J.A.,** Whey proteins protect more than red meat against azoxymethane-induced ACF in Wistar rats, *Cancer Letters,* 2003;198(1): 43-51.

130.**Chia, V., Newcomb, P.A.,** Calcium and colorectal cancer: some questions remain, *Nutrition Reviews,* 2004; 62(3): 115-120.

CHAPTER 8

1.   **Weggemans, R.M., Zock, P.L., and Katan, M.B.,** Dietary cholesterol from eggs increases the ratio of total cholesterol to high-density lipoprotein cholesterol in humans: a meta-analysis, *American Journal of Clinical Nutrition,* 2001;73 (5):885-91.

2.   **Nakamura, Y., Okamura, T., et al,** Egg consumption, serum cholesterol, and cause-specific and all-cause mortality: the National Integrated Project for Prospective Observation of Non-communicable Disease and Its Trends in the Aged, 1980 (NIPPON DATA80), *American Journal of Clinical Nutrition,* 2004; 80(1):58-63.

3.   **Executive summary of the third report of the National Cholesterol Education Program.** Expert panel on detection, evaluation and treatment of high blood cholesterol in adults, *Journal of the American Medical Association, 2001;* 285 (19): 2486-2497.

4.   **Brewer, H.B. Jr.,** Focus on high-density lipoproteins in reducing cardiovascular risk, *American Heart Journal,* 2004;148:S14.

5.   **Fruchart, J-C., Melchior, C., et al,** New risk factors for atherosclerosis and patient risk assessment, *Circulation,* 2004;109: suppl 111:15-19.

6. **Sulcova, J., Hill, M., et al,** Effects of transdermal application of 7-oxo-DHEA on the levels of steroid hormones, gonadotropins and lipids in healthy men, *Physiology Research*, 2001; 50(1): 9-18.

7. **Kalra, D. K.,** Homocysteine and cardiovascular disease, *Current Atherosclerosis Reports*, 2004; 6:101-106.

8. **Montebugnoli, L., Servidio, D., et al,** Poor oral health is associated with coronary heart disease and elevated systemic inflammatory and haemostatic factors, *Journal of Clinical Periodontology*, 2004; 31:25-39.

9. **Sastry, P.S.R.K.,** Occult fungal infection is the underlying pathogenic cause of atherogenesis, *Medical Hypotheses*, 2004; 63: 671-674.

10. **Ridker, P.M, Bassuk, S. S, and Toth, P.,** C-reactive protein and risk of cardiovascular disease: evidence and clinical application, *Current Atherosclerosis Reports* 2003; 5: 341-349.

11. **Ridker, P.M.,** High-sensitivity C-reactive protein, inflammation and cardiovascular risk: from concept to clinical practice to clinical benefit, *American Heart Journal,* 2004; 148(1 Suppl): S19-26.

12. **Jacoby, D.S., Mohler, E.R., and Rader D.J.,** Non-invasive atherosclerosis imaging for predicting cardiovascular events and assessing therapeutic interventions, *Current Atherosclerosis Reports*, 2004; 6: 20-26.

13. **Dubey, R.K., Tofovic, S. P., and Jackson, E.K.,** Cardiovascular pharmacology of estradiol metabolites, *The Journal of Pharmacology and Experimental Therapeutics,* 2004; 308: 403-409.

14. **Larosa, J.C.,** Evidence-based management of dyslipidemias in women, *Current Atherosclerosis Reports* 2003; 5: 379-385.

15. **Hodis, H.N, Mack, W.J, and Lobo, R.,** What is the cardioprotective role of hormone replacement therapy? *Current Atherosclerosis Reports* 2003; 5: 56-66.

16. **Von Eckardstein, A., and Wu, F.C.,** Testosterone and atherosclerosis, *Growth Hormone and IGF-1 Research*, 2003; 13: S72-S84.

17. **Liu, P.Y., Death A.K., Handelsman, D.J.,** Androgens and cardiovascular disease, *Endocrine Reviews,* 2003; 24: 313-340.

18. **Khan S.A., Sane, D.S., et al,** Growth hormone insulin-like growth factor-1 and the aging cardiovascular system, *Cardiovascular Research*, 2002; 54(1): 25-35.

19. **Hoffman R.A., and Ceda G.P.,** Growth hormone and IGF research, IGFs and aging: is there a rationale for hormone replacement therapy? *Growth Hormone and IGF-1 Research,* 2004; 14: 296-300.

20. **Labrie F., Luu-the, V., et al,** Endocrine and intracrine sources of androgens in women: Inhibition of breast cancer and other roles of androgens and their precursor dehydroepiandrosterone, *Endocrine Reviews,* 2003; 24(2): 152-182.

21. **Ng, M.K.C., Nakhla S., et al,** Dehydroepiandrosterone, an adrenal androgen, increases human foam cell formation, *Journal of the American College of Cardiology,* 2003; 42(11): 1967-1974.

22. **Allolio, B., and Arlt, W.,** DHEA treatment: myth or reality, *Trends in Endocrinology and Metabolism,* 2002;13(7): 288-294.

23. **Glueck, C.J., and Streicher, P.,** Cardiovascular and medical ramifications of treatment of subclinical hypothyroidism, *Current Atherosclerosis Reports*, 2003; 5: 73-77.

24. **Guthrie J.R., Taffe, J.R., et al,** Association between hormonal changes at menopause and the risk of a coronary event: a longitudinal study, *Menopause*, 2004;11(3): 315-322.

25. **Imaizumi, M., Akahoshi, M., et al,** Risk for ischemic heart disease and all-cause mortality in subclinical hypothyroidism, *Journal of Clinical Endocrinology and Metabolism*, 2004; 89(7): 3365-3370.

26. **Vivekananthan, D.K., Penn M. S., et al,** Use of antioxidant vitamins for the prevention of cardiovascular disease: meta-analysis of randomised trials, *Lancet,* 2003; 361: 2017-2023.

27. **Kris-Etherton, P.M., Lichtenstein, A.L., et al**, Antioxidant vitamin supplements and cardiovascular disease, *Circulation,* 2004;110: 637-641.

28. **Orbe, J., Rodriguez, R., et al,** Antioxidant vitamins increase the collagen content and reduce MMP-1 in apocrine model of atherosclerosis: implications for plaque stabilization, *Atherosclerosis,* 2003; 167: 45-53.

29. **Tomeo, A.C, Geller, M., et al,** Antioxidant effects of tocotrienols in patients with hyperlipidemia and carotid stenosis-a 2-year experience, *Lipids,* 1995; 30(12): 1179-1183.

30. **Davidson, M.H., and Geohas, C.T.,** Efficacy of over-the-counter nutritional supplements, *Current Atherosclerosis Reports,* 2003; 5: 15-21.

31. **Janikula, M.,** Policosanol: A new treatment for cardiovascular disease, *Alternative Medicine Review,* 2002; 7(3): 203-215.

32. **Kopernik, G., and Shoham, Z.,** Tools for making correct decisions regarding hormone therapy. Part 11. Organ response and clinical applications, *Fertility and Sterility,* 2004; 81(6): 1458 - 1477.

33. **Bowman, R.E., Beck, K.D., Luine, V.N.,** Chronic stress effects on memory: sex differences in performance and monoaminergic activity, *Hormones and Behaviour*, 2003; 43(1): 48-59.

34. **Shaywitz, S.E., Naftolin, F., et al,** Better oral reading and short-term memory in midlife, postmenopausal women taking estrogen, *Menopause,* 2003; 10(5): 120-126.

35. **Galen, B.J., Crooks, V.V., et al,** Hormone use and cognitive performance in women of advanced age, *Journal of the American Geriatric Society,* 2004; 52(2): 182-186.

36. **Kang, J.H., Weuve, J., Grodstein, F.,** Postmenopausal hormone therapy and risk of cognitive decline in community-dwelling aging women, *Neurology,* 2004; 63: 101-107.

37. **Rapp S.R., Espeland, M.A., et al,** Effect of estrogen plus progestin on global cognitive function in postmenopausal women: the Women's Health Initiative memory study: a randomised control trial, *Journal of the American Medical Association,* 2003; 289(20): 2663-2672.

38. **Sherwin, B.B.,** Estrogen and cognitive functioning in women, *Endocrine Reviews,* 2004; 24(2): 133-151.

39. **Schumacher, M., Guennoun, R., et al,** Local synthesis and dual actions of progesterone in the nervous system: neuroprotection and myelination, *Growth Hormone and IGF-1 Research,* 2004; 14: S18-S33.

40. **Azad, N., Pitale, S., et al,** Testosterone treatment enhances regional blood perfusion in hypogonadal men, *Journal of Clinical Endocrinology and Metabolism,* 2003; 88(7): 3064-3068.

41. **Lim, D., Flicker, L., et al,** Can testosterone replacement decrease the memory problem of age? *Medical Hypothesis*, 2003; 60(6): 893-896.

42. **Sherwin, B.B.,** Steroid hormones and cognitive functioning in aging men: a mini review, *Journal of Molecular Neuroscience,* 2003; 20(3): 385-393.

43. **Tan, S.R., and Pu, S, J.,** The andropause and memory loss: is there a link between androgen decline and dementia in the aging male? *Asian Journal of Andrology,* 2001; 3: 169-174.

44. **Trejo, J.L., Carro, E., et al,** Role of serum insulin-like growth factor 1 in mammalian brain aging, *Growth Hormone and IGF -1Research*, 2004; 14: S39-S43.

45. **Hoffman, A.R., and Ceda, G.P.,** IGFs and aging: is there a rationale for hormone replacement therapy? *Growth Hormone and IGF-1 Research,* 2004; 14: 296-300.

46. **Arwert L.I., Deijen, J.B., and Drent, M.L.,** Effects of an oral mixture containing glycine, glutamine and niacin on memory, GH and IGF-1 secretion in middle-aged and elderly subjects, *Nutrition and Neuroscience*, 2003; 6(5): 269-275.

47. **Schumacher, M., Weill-Engerer, S.,** et al, Steroid hormones and neurosteroids in normal and pathological aging of the nervous system, *Progress in Neurobiology*, 2003; 71: 3-29.

48. **Lemon, J.A., Boreham, D.R., and Rollo, C.D.,** A dietary supplement abolishes age-related cognitive decline in transgenic mice expressing elevated free radical processes, *Experimental Biology and Medicine*, 2003; 228: 800-810.

49. **Solomon, P. R., Adams, F.,** et al, Ginkgo for memory enhancement: a randomized controlled trial, *Journal of the American Medical Association*, 2002; 21, 288(7): 835-40.

50. **Stough, C., Lloyd, J.,** et al, The chronic effects of an extract of Bacopa monniera (Brahmi) on cognitive function in healthy human subjects, *Psychopharmacology*, (Berl). 2001; 156(4): 481-484.

51. **Crook, T.H.,** Treatment of age-related cognitive decline: Effects of phosphatidylserine, *Anti-Ageing Medical Therapeutics*, 1998; 2: 20-29.

52. **Messina, M., Gardner, C., and Barnes, S.,** Fourth international symposium on the role of soy in preventing and treating chronic disease, *Journal of Nutrition*, 2002; 132: 547S-551S.

53. **Kreijkamp-Kaspers, S., Kok, L.,** et al, Effect of soy protein containing isoflavones on cognitive function, bone mineral density and plasma lipids in postmenopausal women, a randomised control trial, *Journal of the American Medical Association*, 2004; 292(1): 6-57.

54. **Kritz-Silverstein, D., Von Muhlen, D.,** et al, Isoflavones and cognitive function in older women: the soy and postmenopausal health in aging study, *Menopause*, 2003;10(3): 196-202.

55. **Dijsselbloem, N., Vanden Berghe, W.,** et al, Soy isoflavone phyto-pharmaceuticals in interleukin-6 affections. Multi-purpose nutraceuticals at the crossroad of hormone replacement, anti-cancer and anti-inflammatory therapy, *Biochemical Pharmacology*, 2004; 68: 1171-1185.

56. **Moffat S.D., Zonderman, A.B.,** et al, Free testosterone and risk for Alzheimer's disease in older men, *Neurology*, 2004; 62: 188-193.

57. **Hillen T., Lun A.,** et al, DHEA-S plasma levels and incidence of Alzheimer's disease, *Biological Psychiatry*, 2000; 47(2): 161-163.

58. **Zandi, P.P., James, C.,** et al, Reduced risk of Alzheimer's disease in users of antioxidant vitamin supplements, *Archives of Neurology*, 2004; 61: 82-88.

59. **Morris, D. A, Evans, J, L., et al,** Consumption of Fish and n-3 Fatty Acids and Risk of Incident Alzheimer Disease, *Archives of Neurology,* 2003; 60: 940-946.

60. **Mulnard, R.A., Corrada, M.M., and Kawas, C. H.,** Estrogen replacement therapy, Alzheimer's disease and mild cognitive impairment, *Current Neurology and Neuroscience reports* 2004; 4: 368-373.

61. **Levine A.J., Battista M.,** Estrogen replacement therapy: effects on the cognitive functioning and clinical course of women with Alzheimer's disease, *Archives of Clinical Neuropsychology,* 2004; 19: 769-778.

63. **Tan R. S., and Pu, S.J.,** A pilot study on the effects of testosterone in hypogonadal aging male patients with Alzheimer's disease, *The Aging Male,* 2003; 6(1): 7-13.

64. **Howes, M.J., Perry, N.S., and Houghton, P.J.,** Plants with traditional uses and activities, relevant to the management of Alzheimer's disease and other cognitive disorders, *Phytotherapy Research,* 2003; 17(1): 1-18.

65. **Schwarzschild, M.A., Xu, F., et al,** Neuroprotection by caffeine and more specific A2A receptor antagonists in animal models of Parkinson's disease, *Neurology,* 2003; 61(11 Suppl 6): S55-61.

66. **Muller, T., and Buttner, T., et al,** Coenzyme Q10 supplementation provides mild symptomatic benefit in patients with Parkinson's disease, *Neuroscience Letters,* 2003; 341(3): 201-204.

67. **Coimbra, C.G., and Junqueira, V.B.,** High doses of riboflavin and the elimination of dietary red meat promote the recovery of some motor functions in Parkinson's disease patients, *Brazil Journal of Medical and Biological Research,* 2003; (10): 1409-17.

CHAPTER NINE

1. **Visser, M., Pahor, M., et al,** Relationship of interleukin-6 and tumour necrosis factor-alpha with muscle mass and muscle strength in elderly men and women: The health ABC study, *The Journal of Gerontology,* 2002; 57A, 5; M326-M332.

2. **Bruunsgaard, H., Andersen-Ranberg, K., et al,** Elevated levels of tumour necrosis factor alpha and mortality in centenarians, *American Journal of Medicine,* 2003; 115: 278-283.

3. **Kovacs, E.J., Plackett, T. P., and Witte, P.L.,** Estrogen replacement, aging, and cell-mediated immunity after injury, *Journal of Leukocyte Biology,* 2004; 76: 36-41.

4. **Goodier, M.R., and Imami, N., et al,** Loss of the CD56 hi CD16-NK cell subset and NK cell interferon-gamma production during antiretroviral therapy for HIV-1: partial recovery by growth hormone, *Clinical and Experimental Immunology,* 2003; 134: 470-476.

5. **Napolitano, L.A., Lo, J.C., et al,** Increased thymic mass and circulating naïve CD4 T-cells in HIV-1 infected adults treated with growth hormone, *AIDS,* 2002; 16: 1103-1111.

6. **Silva, C., Zhang, K., et al,** Growth hormone prevents human immunodeficiency virus-induced neuronal p53 expression, *Annals of Neurology,* 2003; 54: 605-614.

7. **Fawzi. W.W., Gernard, P.H., et al,** A randomised trial of multivitamin supplements and HIV disease progression and mortality, *New England Journal of Medicine,* 2004; 351; (1): 23-32.

8. **Allard, J.P., Aghdassi, E., et al,** Effects of vitamin E and C supplementation on oxidative stress and viral load in HIV-infected subjects, *AIDS,* 1998; 12(13): 1653-1659.

9. **Jaruga, P., Jaruga, B., et al,** Supplementation with antioxidant vitamins prevents oxidative modification of DNA in lymphocytes of HIV-infected patients, *Free Radical Biology and Medicine,* 2002; 32(5): 414-420.

10. **Lopez, O., Bonnefont-Rousselot, D., et al,** Could antioxidant supplementation reduce antiretroviral therapy-induced chronic stable hyperlactatemia, *Biomedicine and Pharmacotherapy,* 2003;57: 113-116.

11. **Patrick, L.,** Nutrients and HIV: Part 2-Vitamins A and E, Zinc, B-Vitamins, and Magnesium, *Alternative Medicine Review* 2000; 5(1): 39-48.

12. **Rayman, M.P.,** The argument for increasing selenium intake, *Proceedings of the Nutrition Society,* 2002; 61: 203-215.

13. **Kupka, R., and Msamanga, G.I., et al,** Selenium status is associated with accelerated HIV disease progression among HIV-1 infected pregnant women in Tanzania, *Journal of Nutrition,* 2004; 134: 2556-2560.

14. **Fawzi, W.,** Micronutrients and human immunodeficiency virus type 1 disease progression among adults and children, *Clinical Infectious Diseases* 2003; 37(Suppl 2): S112-116.

15. **Vanderhaeghe, L.R., and Bouic, P.J.,** The immune system cure, New York: Kensington, 1999.

16. **Offner, H.,** Neuroimmunoprotective effects of estrogen and derivatives in experimental autoimmune encephalomyelitis: Therapeutic implications for multiple sclerosis, *Journal of Neuroscience Research,* 2004; 78: 603-624.

17. **Palaszynski, K.M., Liu, H., et al,** Estriol treatment ameliorates disease in males with experimental autoimmune encephalomyelitis: implications for multiple sclerosis, *Journal of Neuroimmunology,* 2004; 149(1-2): 84-89.

18. **Palaszynski, K.M., Loo, K.K., et al,** Androgens are protective in experimental autoimmune encephalomyelitis: implications for multiple sclerosis, *Journal of Neuroimmunology,* 2004; 146: 144-152.

19. **Fernandez, M., Giuliani, A., et al,** Thyroid hormone administration enhances remyelination in chronic demyelinating inflammatory disease, *Proceeds of the National Academy of Science* USA, 2004; 101(46): 163-638.

20. **Van Amerongen, B.M., Dijkstra, C.D., et al,** Multiple sclerosis and vitamin D: an update, *European Journal of Clinical Nutrition,* 2004; 58: 1095-1109.

21. **Wade, D.T., Young, C.A., et al,** Randomised placebo controlled exploratory study of vitamin B-12, lofepramine, and L-phenylalanine (the "Cari Loder regime") in the treatment of multiple sclerosis, *Journal of Neurology, Neurosurgery and Psychiatry,* 2002; 73: 246-249.

22. **Morini, M., Roccatagliata, L., et al,** Alpha-lipoic acid is effective in prevention and treatment of experimental autoimmune encephalomyelitis, *Journal of Neuroimmunology,* 2004; 148(1-2): 146-153.

23. **Nordvik, I., Myhr, K. M., et al,** Effect of dietary advice and n-3 supplementation in newly diagnosed MS patients, *Acta Neurologica Scandanavia,* 2000; 102(3): 143-149.

CHAPTER 10:

1. **Sator, P-G., Rabe, T., and Zouboulis C.C.,** Skin aging and sex hormones in women-clinical perspectives for intervention by hormone replacement therapy. *Experimental Dermatology* 2004; 13 (Suppl 4): 36-40.

2. **Brincat, M.P.,** Hormone replacement therapy and the skin, *Maturitas,* 2000; 35: 107117.

3. **Chiu, A., and Kimball, A.B.,** Topical vitamins, minerals and botanic ingredients as modulators of environmental and chronological skin damage, *British Journal of Dermatology* 2003;149: 681-691.

4. **Humbert, P.G., Haftek, M., et al,** Topical ascorbic acid on photoaged skin.Clinical, topographical and ultrastructural evaluation: double blind study vs. placebo, *Experimental Dermatology*, 2003; 12: 237-244.

5. **Chiu, A., and Kimball, A.B.,** Topical vitamins, minerals and botanic ingredients as modulators of environmental and chronological skin damage, *British Journal of Dermatology,* 2003; 149: 681-691.

7. **Breitner, H.,** Randomized placebo-controlled, double blind study on the clinical efficacy of a cream containing 5% alpha-lipoic acid related to photoageing of facial skin, *British Journal of Dermatology,* 2003; 149: 841-849.

8. **Uhoda I., Faska, N., et al,** Split face study on the cutaneous tensile effect of 2-dimethylaminoethanol (deanol) gel, *Skin Research Technology,* 2002; 8(3): 164-167.

9. **Janowiak, J.J., and Ham, C.,** Practitioners guide to hair loss Part 1- History, biology, genetics, prevention, conventional treatments and herbals, *Alternative and Complementary Therapies* 2004; 10(3): 135-143.

10. **Hoffmann, R., Niiyama, S., et al,** 17 alpha-estradiol induces aromatase activity in intact human anagen hair follicles ex vivo, *Experimental Dermatology,* 2002; 11(4): 376-380.

11. **Lindenbaum, E.S., Feitelberg, A.L., et al,** Pilot study of a novel treatment for androgenetic alopecia using enriched cell culture medium: clinical trials, *Dermatology Online Journal,* 2003; 9(1): 4-20.

12. **Prager, N., Bickett, K., et al,** A randomised, double-blind, placebo-controlled trial to determine the effectiveness of botanically derived inhibitors of 5-alpha-reductase in the treatment of androgenetic alopecia, *The Journal of Alternative and Complementary Medicine* 2002; 8(2): 143-152.

13. **Perez, H.B.S.,** Ketaconazole as an adjunct to finasteride in the treatment of androgenetic alopecia in men, *Medical Hypotheses,* 2004; 62:112-115.

14. **Takahashi, T., Kamimura, A., et al,** The first clinical trial of topical application of procyanidin B-2 to investigate its potential as a hair growing agent, *Phytotherapy Research,* 2001; 15(4):331-336.

CHAPTER 11:

1. **Fenech, M.,** Nutritional treatment of genome instability: a paradigm shift in disease prevention and in the setting of recommended dietary allowance, *Nutrition Research Reviews,* 2003; 16: 109-122.

INDEX